THE QUALITY MINDSET IN HEALTHCARE

WHY SAFETY, TRUST, AND EFFECTIVE CARE BEGIN WITH HOW WE THINK

SRAVAN KUMAR NIDIGANTI

notionpress.com

INDIA • SINGAPORE • MALAYSIA

ISBN
Paperback 979-8-90342-681-2
Hardcase 979-8-90479-880-2

Contents

Foreword

Why This Book Matters Now

Healthcare is changing faster than ever before. Systems are becoming more automated, decisions are more data-driven, and expectations are higher on all sides. In the midst of this transformation, quality is often discussed as a function, something that can be measured, audited, optimized, or certified. Yet what is frequently missing from these conversations is the human reality of healthcare and the mindset required to protect it.

This book arrives at an important moment.

Quality challenges today are rarely caused by lack of intelligence, skill or effort. They emerge from complexity, speed and disconnected decision-making. As healthcare ecosystems grow more complicated, the consequences of shallow quality thinking grow deeper. The need is no longer just for people who know how to execute quality tasks, but for professionals who know how to **think in quality terms**—across systems, across time and across human impact.

What makes this book distinctive is that it does not attempt to teach quality as a checklist or framework. Instead, it invites the reader to see quality as a responsibility and a way of thinking. Drawing from real-world experience across healthcare quality, healthcare IT, patient safety, and leadership, it connects everyday decisions to the lived experiences of patients and members.

This is not a book about perfection. It is a book about awareness. It is written for those who want to do more than comply, for those who want to protect access, safety, dignity, and trust in an increasingly complex healthcare environment.

If you work in healthcare quality, operations, technology, leadership, or policy, this book will challenge how you see your role. And if you carry its mindset forward, it will quietly influence decisions long after the final page.

Preface

Why I Wrote This Book

I did not set out to write a book about healthcare quality. This book grew out of questions that kept returning, no matter how much experience I gained or how many systems I worked with.

Why do quality issues keep surfacing even when skilled people do everything right?

Why do systems that pass validation still confuse the people they are meant to serve?

Why does healthcare sometimes feel efficient on the inside and overwhelming on the outside?

Over years of working in healthcare quality, healthcare IT, patient safety, and operational environments, and through my academic journey in healthcare administration, I began to see a pattern. Quality failures were rarely due to a lack of knowledge or effort. They were about mindset. They were about how decisions were framed, how assumptions were made, and how responsibility was defined.

I wrote this book because I believe healthcare quality professionals are often underestimated by organizations and sometimes by themselves. We are positioned as checkers at the end of processes, when in reality we sit at the center of decisions that shape access, safety, affordability, and trust. We influence outcomes for people we may never meet, often without recognition, and sometimes without authority.

This book is written in the first person because it reflects what I have seen, learned, and questioned along the way. It blends experience with research, reflection with reality. It is intentionally written in plain language because quality should be understood, not hidden behind jargon.

You won't find step-by-step instructions here. Instead, you'll find perspective. This book is meant to slow you down just enough to think differently, to see the system more clearly, and to recognize the quiet power of your role.

If this book changes how you approach even one decision, it will have done its job.

Acknowledgments

Those Who Shaped the Thinking Behind This Work

No book like this is written alone, even when one name appears on the cover. This work has been shaped by countless conversations, challenges, and shared experiences across years in healthcare quality and leadership.

I am deeply grateful to the colleagues and teams I have worked alongside, those in healthcare quality, operations, healthcare IT, patient safety, and clinical support, who brought dedication, curiosity, and integrity to complex work. Many of the lessons in this book came not from success, but from thoughtful discussions after things did not go as planned.

I also acknowledge all my leaders and mentors, especially my executive coach, **Pradeepa Narayanaswamy**, for being such an inspiration who demonstrates, sometimes quietly, what it means to prioritize people over speed, understanding over convenience, and long-term trust over short-term wins. Their influence reinforced the idea that quality is ultimately a leadership responsibility.

My academic journey in healthcare administration further shaped this work. The discipline of research, evidence-based thinking and ethical reflection deepened my understanding of how systems behave and how change must be grounded in both data and humanity.

Finally, I thank my Spouse, **Srideepika Nidiganti**; my Son, **Veda Sricharan Nidiganti**; my Parents; family and friends for their encouragement and support. Healthcare quality work often happens in invisible spaces, but it requires visible commitment. Their encouragement made it possible to reflect, write, and complete this book.

This book is the result of shared learning, even when the words are my own.

CHAPTER 1

The Healthcare Ecosystem: Seeing the Whole Before Fixing the Part

When people talk about healthcare, they often describe it as if it were a place: a hospital, a clinic, a pharmacy, a doctor's office. Those are the visible touchpoints, so it makes sense. But after spending years working across healthcare quality, healthcare IT, patient safety, and operational environments, I have learned that healthcare is not a place at all. It is a system. More accurately, it is an ecosystem.

I start this book here because many quality challenges don't come from lack of effort or lack of expertise. They come from something far more subtle: **not fully seeing the system we are working inside of**. When we focus only on our immediate task or domain, we miss how decisions travel, how assumptions compound, and how small choices ripple outward until they reach a real person.

Early in my career, I believed that doing my part well was enough. If I validated what I was assigned, followed requirements carefully, and met timelines, quality would naturally follow. That belief worked in theory, but it did not survive real healthcare.

Over time, I began noticing a pattern. Systems were behaving exactly as designed, yet members were confused. Policies were followed correctly, yet access was delayed. Changes were deployed successfully, yet trust eroded downstream. From the inside, everything looked compliant. From the outside, quality felt absent. That disconnect forced me to rethink what quality really means in healthcare.

Healthcare today is one of the most complex ecosystems in existence. It includes patients and members, providers and caregivers, health plans, clinical programs, pharmacies, manufacturers, healthcare IT platforms, data systems, regulatory bodies, and vendors, all interacting constantly. Each part depends on the others, and none of them operates in isolation. A change in one area rarely stays contained. It travels.

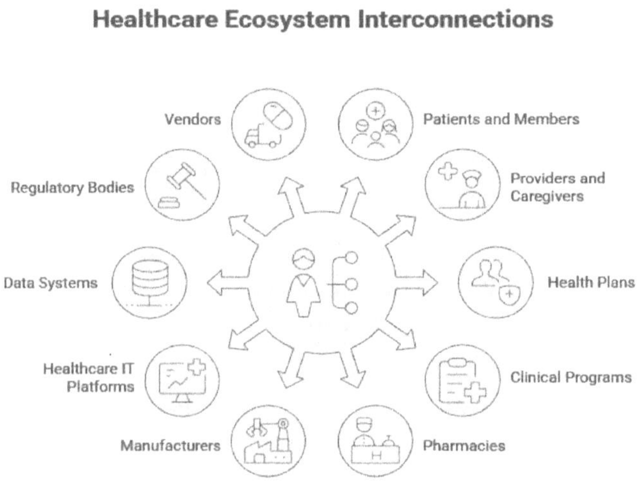

What I have seen repeatedly is that **quality problems rarely originate where they are felt**. They originate earlier, often quietly at points where decisions are interpreted, translated into system logic, or handed off between teams. By the time the issue reaches a member, it has already passed through multiple layers of the ecosystem.

This is where healthcare quality professionals truly sit, not at the end, but in the middle. We operate at the intersection of policy and practice, technology and behavior, speed and safety. Even when our role is defined narrowly, the impact of our decisions is not.

One of the most important realizations in my career was understanding that healthcare systems do not think. They execute. They apply rules, logic and workflows exactly as designed. They do not question intent. They do not recognize stress or urgency. They do not understand the difference between inconvenience and harm. Once a decision is automated, it scales instantly.

That is both the strength and the risk of modern healthcare.

More than 70 percent of healthcare interactions today involve digital systems in some way. Administrative complexity alone is estimated to cost the US healthcare system between **$250 and $300 billion each year**. These numbers are often discussed as efficiency problems, but what they really represent are delayed decisions, repeated explanations, avoidable confusion, and unnecessary stress for people who are already navigating illness or uncertainty.

Quality professionals exist to reduce that burden, even when we never see it directly.

One way I often explain the healthcare ecosystem is this: a need enters the system, but an experience comes out. Between those two points sit eligibility rules, clinical criteria, system logic, workflows, integrations, and human judgment. Each step introduces the possibility of friction or clarity. Quality lives in how smoothly that journey unfolds.

What makes this difficult is that many quality risks are invisible from within a single domain. A decision that looks reasonable in isolation can create unintended consequences when combined with timing, scale, or real-world behavior. I have seen small assumptions made in good faith lead to large downstream impact simply because no one paused to ask how the decision would behave once it left the room.

"Every system is perfectly designed to get the results it gets."

When outcomes create confusion, delay or harm, the issue is rarely effort. It is designed.

Some of the most effective healthcare organizations I have worked with understand this intuitively. They involve quality early, not as a final checkpoint, but as a thinking partner. They encourage questions instead of rushing to certainty. They look at changes through a member-impact lens, not just a system-readiness checklist. They test beyond ideal scenarios and treat access and affordability as quality outcomes, not operational side effects.

These are not complex practices. They are mindset-driven practices.

Healthcare is evolving quickly. In the past, systems were fragmented and heavily manual. Today, platforms are integrated and automated. Tomorrow, decisions will increasingly be assisted, or even initiated, by artificial intelligence. As this evolution continues, the consequences of poor design will scale faster than ever before.

That is why understanding the healthcare ecosystem is no longer optional for quality professionals. It is foundational.

Quality is not about fixing broken parts after the fact. It is about understanding how the whole system behaves before harm occurs. Once you begin to see healthcare this way, your role changes. Your questions change. Your sense of responsibility deepens.

Before moving forward, I invite you to pause and reflect. Do you understand how your work connects to the broader healthcare ecosystem? Where do decisions hand off from your area to another? Who experiences the outcome of your work first? What assumptions do you make so often that you no longer notice them?

These questions are not meant to create doubt. They are meant to create awareness.

Because awareness is where quality truly begins.

CHAPTER 2

Healthcare Quality: What We Are Really Protecting

For many years, healthcare quality was explained to me through metrics: accuracy rates, compliance scores, turnaround times, defect counts, and audit findings. Anyone who has worked in quality knows these measures well, and they serve an important purpose. They tell us how systems perform. But the longer I worked in healthcare—and the more stories I heard from members, providers, and frontline teams—the more I realized something was missing.

Those measures describe performance.
They do not describe experience.
And healthcare quality lives in the space between the two.

When someone seeks care, they are not thinking about process maturity models or control effectiveness. They are thinking about whether help will arrive in time, whether it will make sense, whether it will be affordable, and whether it will make their situation better—or worse. Quality exists or fails in those moments. Everything else is infrastructure built to support them.

One of the most important shifts in my thinking came when I stopped asking, *"Did this meet requirements?"* and started asking, *"What are we actually protecting here?"* The answer was never just compliance. We were protecting safety, access, dignity, affordability, trust, often without explicitly naming them.

Healthcare quality is not a single attribute. It is a balance of responsibilities that constantly pull against one another. Over time, I have seen organizations excel in one area while unintentionally weakening another. Speed improves, but clarity disappears. Controls tighten, but access suffers. Automation increases consistency, but equity gaps widen. None of this happens because people don't care. It happens because quality is treated as a target instead of a balance.

Safety is usually the first word that comes up in quality conversations, and rightly so. But safety in modern healthcare is broader than preventing clinical errors. It includes preventing delays that worsen conditions, preventing confusion that leads people to abandon care, and preventing financial stress that forces unsafe choices. I have seen situations where no clinical error occurred, yet the outcome was still unsafe because the system created fear, delay, or uncertainty. In those moments, safety was already compromised—even if no incident report was ever filed.

Effectiveness is often misunderstood as technical correctness. But in real healthcare, effectiveness means that care actually reaches the person who needs it and improves their situation. A decision can be evidence-based, policy-aligned, and system-approved, and still be ineffective if it never results in timely, usable care. Industry research shows that a significant portion of recommended care is never followed, often due to access barriers, confusion, or cost. That is not a patient failure. It is a quality failure.

Timeliness looks simple on paper and becomes complex in practice. From a system perspective, a delay of a few days may seem acceptable. From a human perspective, waiting carries emotional weight. Anxiety grows, conditions worsen, trust erodes. I have seen healthcare systems move quickly internally while members waited weeks for clarity. Internally, everything looked efficient. Externally, quality felt absent. Timeliness must always be judged from the experience of the person waiting—not from the comfort of the system processing.

Efficiency is often framed as cost reduction, but in quality work, inefficiency usually signals poor design. Rework, escalations, repeated calls, and manual overrides do not happen because people are careless. They happen because systems were not built with real-world behavior in mind. Studies estimate that administrative inefficiencies account for roughly a quarter to a third of US healthcare spending. Reducing this waste is not just a financial goal; it is a quality responsibility, because inefficiency steals time, energy, and trust from people who are already vulnerable.

Equity has become impossible to ignore in healthcare quality, and for good reason. Systems often work well for people who fit the "standard" scenario—those with stable coverage, digital access, health literacy, and flexibility. But quality must also work for people who don't fit that mold. When processes assume perfect understanding or ideal conditions, they unintentionally disadvantage those who need care the most. Equity is not achieved through good intent alone. It requires deliberate quality thinking at every decision point.

Patient-centeredness is sometimes described as a soft concept, but in practice, it is one of the strongest indicators of whether quality will hold. When systems are designed without considering how real people navigate illness, stress, and uncertainty, cracks appear immediately. A member-centered system does not remove rules or boundaries. It explains them clearly, applies them consistently, and respects the dignity of the person affected. When that doesn't happen, people disengage—and disengagement is often the earliest warning sign of quality failure.

Trust is the outcome that ties all of these dimensions together. Trust is built when systems behave predictably, explanations make sense, and outcomes feel fair—even when the answer is not what someone hoped for. Trust is fragile. Once broken, it is difficult to restore. Research consistently shows that loss of trust leads to delayed care, reduced adherence, and higher long-term costs. In healthcare, trust is not an abstract value. It is a measurable driver of outcomes.

Over time, I have come to see healthcare quality not as a checklist of attributes, but as a continuous balancing act. Every decision shifts that balance slightly. Every assumption carries weight. Every shortcut, however small, compounds at scale. Quality professionals are not just enforcing standards. We are shaping experiences—often invisibly.

Quality is not measured by how well systems work,
But by how safely people live within them.

Evolving Healthcare Quality

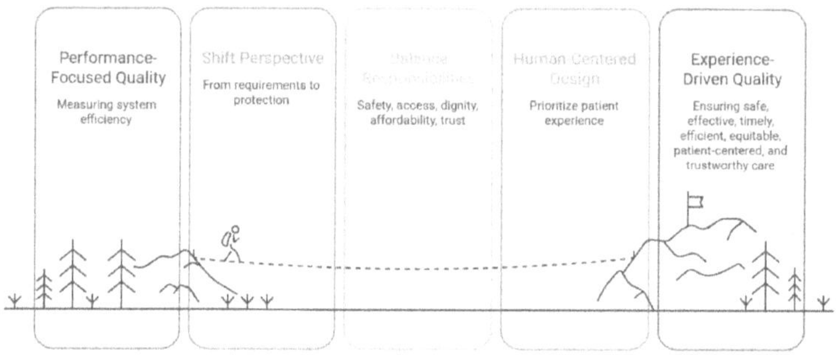

This chapter exists to anchor the rest of the book in a simple truth: healthcare quality is not theoretical. It is lived. It shows up in access to care, in financial burden, in clarity of communication, and in whether people feel supported or abandoned by the system.

In the chapters that follow, we will go deeper into each of these dimensions one by one, not as isolated concepts, but as lived responsibilities. We will explore what they mean in real healthcare, how they break down, how they are measured, and how they must evolve—especially in a world increasingly shaped by technology and AI.

As you continue reading, I invite you to reflect not on how well you execute tasks, but on how your decisions influence people you may never meet. That perspective—quiet, human, and responsibility-driven—is the foundation of a true quality mindset.

Before moving forward, pause for a moment.

Where in your work do you define quality too narrowly?

Where do you feel tension between speed, cost and care?

What would change if you viewed quality not as a requirement to meet, but as a responsibility to protect?

Those questions will guide everything that follows.

Moment That Changed My Thinking: The Day Everything Was "Correct," But Still Wrong

Early in my healthcare career, we deployed a system update that passed every checkpoint.

- Requirements were validated.
- Test cases were executed.
- Approvals were signed.
- Metrics were green.

From the inside, it was a success.

A few weeks later, call volume began rising. Not dramatically, just enough to notice. Members were confused about benefit details. Nothing was technically incorrect. The logic was functioning exactly as designed. But people were struggling to understand what had changed.

I remember reviewing the configuration and thinking, *The system is right.*

But then, I asked a different question: *Is the experience right?*

That moment unsettled me. For the first time, I saw clearly that compliance does not guarantee clarity. Correctness does not guarantee quality. And validation does not guarantee understanding.

That was the day I stopped asking – **"Did we meet requirements?"**

and started asking – **"What will this feel like to someone who doesn't sit in this room?"**

That shift changed my leadership permanently.

CHAPTER 3

Patient Safety: How We Actually Protect People, Not Just Report Harm

As my understanding of patient safety matured, I also began to see tools differently. Early on, safety tools were introduced to me as formal exercises we did after something went wrong. Root cause analyses were conducted. Action plans were documented. Lessons learned were shared. On paper, it all looked thorough.

But, over time, I realized that tools don't create safety. They reflect how seriously an organization takes it.

Take root cause analysis, for example. In theory, it exists to understand why harm occurred. In practice, I have seen it used in two very different ways. In one environment, it became a mechanism to identify where an individual failed. The conclusions were predictable, and so were the outcomes: training reminders, policy reinforcement, and eventually repetition of the same issues. In another environment, the same tool was used to examine system design, assumptions, and conditions. The conversations were uncomfortable, but the outcomes were different. Processes changed, hand-offs improved, and signals surfaced earlier the next time.

The tool was the same. The mindset was not.

I have learned that patient safety tools are only as effective as the questions we are willing to ask. When we ask, "Who made the mistake?" learning stops. When we ask, "What made this outcome possible?" prevention begins.

Failure Mode and Effects Analysis taught me a similar lesson. On paper, it is a proactive safety tool—designed to identify where things *might* go wrong before they do. But I have seen it reduced to a compliance activity, completed quickly to satisfy a requirement. When that happens, the exercise loses its power.

The most effective uses of proactive safety tools I have seen were grounded in imagination and humility. Teams asked what happens when information is incomplete, when timing doesn't align, and when people are under stress. They didn't assume ideal conditions. They assumed reality. And because of that, they uncovered risks that would never appear in retrospective reviews.

That shift, from ideal design to realistic design, is one of the most powerful patient safety practices I know.

Incident and near-miss reporting is another area where mindset matters more than mechanics. Many organizations struggle with underreporting, and the reasons are rarely technical. People don't report when they fear blame, when they believe nothing will change, or when reporting feels like self-exposure.

I have seen environments where near misses were treated as failures, and environments where they were treated as gifts. In the latter, reporting increased, not because people were making more mistakes, but because they trusted the system to learn rather than punish. Those organizations identified patterns earlier and intervened sooner. Safety improved not because people were more careful, but because systems became more honest.

Honesty is one of the most underrated patient safety practices.

Some of the most meaningful safety improvements I have witnessed came from listening to signals that were not officially labeled as safety issues at all. Repeated questions from patients, confusion about next steps, escalations that felt routine, and delays that were technically within acceptable timeframes but emotionally distressing.

When quality teams treat these signals as noise, risk accumulates quietly. When they treat them as early warnings, harm is often prevented before it occurs. Patient safety lives in these early moments, long before something becomes reportable.

In US healthcare, research consistently shows that communication failures are among the leading contributors to unsafe outcomes. Studies suggest that over half of serious adverse events involve some form of breakdown in communication or coordination. That reality has reshaped how I think about safety. It is not just about preventing errors, it is about ensuring understanding—between systems, between teams, and between healthcare and the people it serves.

Clear communication is a safety intervention.

Technology has complicated patient safety in new ways. Electronic systems have improved legibility, standardization, and data availability. But they have also introduced new risks—alert fatigue, overreliance on automation, and loss of situational awareness. I have seen safety events occur not because systems failed, but because humans trusted them too much or did not fully understand their limitations.

This is where modern patient safety requires a new kind of thinking. We can no longer ask only whether a system is accurate. We must ask whether it is understandable, interruptible, and resilient. Safety in automated environments depends on how well systems support human judgment, not how perfectly they execute logic.

The most forward-thinking safety practices I have seen today involve continuous monitoring rather than episodic review. Organizations are paying attention to trends instead of waiting for incidents. They look at patterns in access delays, repeated overrides, escalation frequency, and user behavior. These signals don't replace traditional safety reviews, but they extend safety upstream, where prevention is still possible.

As artificial intelligence becomes more common in healthcare workflows, patient safety will face both opportunities and risks. AI can detect patterns humans might miss, it can surface early warning signals, but it can also obscure decision-making and scale bias if quality thinking is not embedded from the start.

The future of patient safety will depend on who is involved in design decisions, not just who reviews outcomes. Quality professionals must be present early, asking how systems behave when assumptions fail and how people experience decisions made by algorithms they do not see.

This is why patient safety, more than any other quality dimension, reinforces the truth that runs through this book. Mastering tools does not achieve safety. Tools are important, but they are not enough. Safety is achieved by a mindset that prioritizes prevention over explanation, curiosity over certainty, and people over processes.

Patient safety is not something we turn on when something goes wrong.

It is something we practice every time we design, decide, or deploy.

And, when safety is treated as a mindset, harm is prevented quietly—before it ever needs a name.

Mindset in Action

In healthcare, patient safety is often approached as a discipline of response. Something happens, an incident is logged, an investigation follows, and corrective actions are assigned. From a skillset perspective, this feels complete. The right steps are taken. The right tools are used. The process moves forward.

But, over time, I have learned that safety rarely fails in the moment an incident occurs. It fails much earlier—when assumptions go unquestioned, when confusion is normalized, and when silence is mistaken for stability.

A skillset-driven approach to safety focuses on detecting and fixing errors after harm becomes visible. It measures how well teams respond once something has gone wrong. That approach is necessary, but it is incomplete. It treats safety as an event rather than a condition.

A mindset-driven approach to safety begins with a different question: *What conditions make harm more likely before anyone notices?* It pays attention to early signals—repeated questions, small delays, workarounds that quietly become routine. It recognizes that people adapt to systems, and that those adaptations often carry risk.

In one healthcare environment, a recurring pattern emerged that never appeared in incident reports. Members were calling multiple times with the same questions, expressing uncertainty about next steps. From a performance standpoint, nothing was broken. Calls were answered, decisions were accurate, and timelines were technically met. From a safety mindset, something was clearly wrong. Confusion was accumulating, and confusion is a known precursor to harm.

Instead of waiting for an adverse event to validate concern, quality leaders stepped in early. They examined how information was delivered, how expectations were set, and how silence between steps was interpreted. Small design changes were made—clearer explanations, better sequencing, explicit timelines. No incident ever occurred. Nothing dramatic happened. But harm was prevented.

That outcome would not have been possible through skill alone. It required a mindset—the willingness to treat uncertainty as risk, to see confusion as a safety signal, and to act before harm demanded attention.

This is what mindset in action looks like. It is quieter than a response, less visible than a correction, but far more powerful.

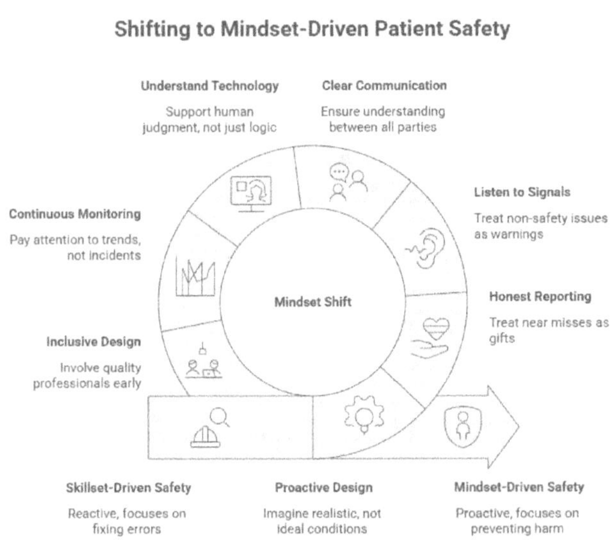
Shifting to Mindset-Driven Patient Safety
Understand Technology
Support human judgment, not just logic
Clear Communication
Ensure understanding between all parties
Listen to Signals
Treat non-safety issues as warnings
Continuous Monitoring
Pay attention to trends, not incidents
Mindset Shift
Honest Reporting
Treat near misses as gifts
Inclusive Design
Involve quality professionals early
Skillset-Driven Safety
Reactive, focuses on fixing errors
Proactive Design
Imagine realistic, not ideal conditions
Mindset-Driven Safety
Proactive, focuses on preventing harm

When quality is treated as a skillset, safety is something we fix. When quality is treated as a mindset, safety is something we protect.

And that difference, between fixing and protecting, is where healthcare quality truly resides.

CHAPTER 4

Effectiveness: When Care Actually Makes a Difference

For a long time, I thought effectiveness in healthcare was straightforward. If care followed evidence-based guidelines, aligned with policy, and met clinical standards, it was effective. That definition looked clean on paper. It also didn't survive contact with reality.

What changed my thinking was watching how often "right" care failed to change outcomes, not because the science was wrong, but because the system couldn't translate intent into action. Effectiveness, I learned, is not proven when a decision is made. It is proven only when care reaches a person in a way they can use, trust and sustain.

In healthcare, effectiveness is not about correctness alone; it is about impact.

I have seen care plans that were clinically sound fall apart because timing didn't align with real life. I have seen evidence-based recommendations go unused because they arrived without clarity or context. I have seen people labeled as non-adherent when, in truth, the system never made adherence realistic. None of these situations reflected a lack of medical knowledge. They reflected a gap between design and lived experience.

Effectiveness fails quietly when systems assume ideal behavior.

In the United States, research consistently shows that a significant portion of recommended care never translates into action. Estimates suggest that roughly **20 percent of patients do not receive recommended evidence-based care**, while another **20–30 percent** do not follow treatment plans as intended. These numbers are often discussed as compliance issues, but through a quality lens, they reveal something deeper. Care that cannot be acted upon is not effective, regardless of how well it was designed.

What I have come to understand is that effectiveness lives at the intersection of science and context. Evidence tells us what should work. Systems determine whether it actually does.

One of the most common threats to effectiveness is fragmentation. Care decisions are made in one place, executed in another, and experienced somewhere else entirely. Information moves through systems, teams, and technologies that do not always share the same assumptions or priorities. By the time care reaches the patient or member, pieces are missing, or meaning has been lost.

When effectiveness breaks, it rarely breaks loudly. It shows up as missed follow-ups, incomplete care journeys, and outcomes that fall short of expectations. From the system's perspective, care was offered. From the person's perspective, it never fully arrived.

Quality work in effectiveness begins with asking a simple but powerful question: *What happens after this decision leaves us?*

Over time, I learned to see effectiveness not as a single moment, but as a chain. Each link matters. Evidence selection, Translation into policy, System configuration, Communication, Timing, Support, Follow-through. A weakness at any point can break the chain, even if every individual step appears correct.

This is where quality tools are often introduced—measures of outcomes, adherence rates, gap-in-care analyses, and performance indicators. These tools are valuable, but only when they are used to understand why care is not working, not just to report that it isn't. I have seen effectiveness metrics used to pressure teams to improve numbers without addressing underlying barriers. When that happens, performance may improve temporarily, but outcomes rarely do.

The most effective use of measurement I have seen focuses on learning, not enforcement. Teams look for patterns rather than exceptions. They ask where people drop off and why. They examine whether systems are enabling action or simply issuing recommendations.

Effectiveness improves when curiosity replaces judgment.

Technology has played a major role in shaping modern effectiveness. Clinical decision support, automated reminders and digital pathways have made it easier to scale evidence-based care. But technology has also exposed a hard truth: reminding someone to do something does not mean they can.

I have seen systems generate perfectly timed reminders that ignored affordability, access, or understanding. From a technical standpoint, the system worked. From a human standpoint, effectiveness still failed. Technology can amplify evidence, but it cannot substitute for empathy or context.

As healthcare increasingly turns to artificial intelligence, effectiveness will be shaped by new possibilities and new risks. AI can identify care gaps earlier, personalize recommendations, and predict outcomes more accurately than ever before. Used thoughtfully, it can close the gap between evidence and action. Used carelessly, it can widen it—especially if recommendations are optimized for averages rather than individuals.

AI does not define effectiveness. It reflects the priorities we built into it.

The future of effectiveness will depend less on how advanced our tools become and more on whether we design systems that respect human reality. Care must be understandable. It must be timely. It must be feasible. And it must be supported in ways that recognize that people are navigating health alongside work, family, fear, and uncertainty.

This is where effectiveness becomes a mindset issue.

When effectiveness is treated as a skillset, the focus stays on execution—following guidelines, closing gaps, meeting targets. When it is treated as a mindset, the focus shifts to outcomes—asking whether care truly made a difference in someone's life. That shift changes how decisions are made, how systems are designed, and how success is defined.

I no longer ask only whether care was evidence-based. I ask whether it was reachable, understandable, and sustainable. I ask whether the system supported action or issued instructions. I ask whether effectiveness was designed or merely assumed.

Effectiveness is not achieved by doing the right thing once. It is achieved by designing systems that help people do the right thing over time.

And, when effectiveness is approached with that mindset, quality moves beyond compliance and becomes something far more meaningful: a force that actually improves lives.

Mindset in Action

Effectiveness in healthcare is often treated as a moment of confirmation. Evidence is followed, guidelines are applied, and the recommendation is correct. From a skillset perspective, the work feels complete once the decision is made and documented.

But effectiveness does not live at the moment of decision. It lives at the moment of use.

A mindset-driven approach to effectiveness forces us to follow care beyond the point of approval and into real life. It asks whether someone could act on what was recommended, whether the timing made sense, whether the path forward was clear, and whether the system supported follow-through, rather than assuming it.

In one healthcare environment, preventive care recommendations were generated accurately and consistently. Yet outcomes remained unchanged. When quality teams looked beyond the recommendation itself, they discovered that people understood *what* was being asked but not *how* to act on it. Appointments were hard to schedule, costs were unclear, and next steps were vague. Once those barriers were addressed, effectiveness improved—without changing the clinical guidance at all.

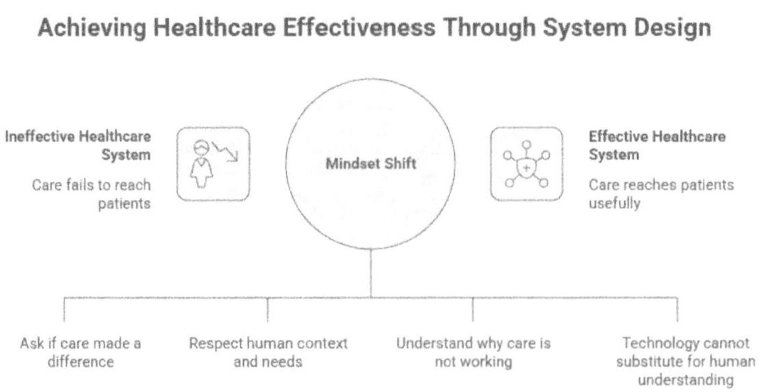

When quality is treated as a skillset, effectiveness is confirmed at the point of correctness.

When quality is treated as a mindset, effectiveness is proven at the point of impact.

Moment That Changed My Thinking: The Near Miss No One Reported

In my research on end-to-end healthcare system quality, I came across an instance in which a team conducted a routine review of incident reports in one environment. The data showed minimal safety issues. On paper, it looked stable.

But something felt off.

Frontline teams were frequently escalating cases, not as incidents, but as "clarifications." Members were calling multiple times to confirm next steps. Nothing had officially gone wrong, yet tension was building beneath the surface.

When we looked deeper, we realized that confusion was acting as a precursor to harm. The system wasn't failing loudly. It was drifting quietly.

No adverse event had occurred.

No formal error had been logged.

But safety was already weakening.

We adjusted the timing of communication, simplified explanations and clarified transitional steps. No headline event followed, and nothing dramatic.

But the volume of escalations declined.

The repeated calls stopped.

The silence felt different.

That moment taught me something profound:

Safety does not begin with incident reports.

It begins with curiosity.

And prevention is invisible—by design.

CHAPTER 5

Patient-Centeredness: Designing Quality Through the Human Experience

For a long time, patient-centeredness was described to me as a communication skill. Listen better. Explain more clearly. Be empathetic. Those ideas are important, but they barely scratch the surface of what patient-centeredness truly means in healthcare. Over time, I learned that patient-centeredness is not something we add to healthcare after it is built. It is something we either design into systems from the beginning or struggle to retrofit later.

Patient-centeredness is not about being nice; it is about being intentional.

I began to understand this when I noticed how often healthcare systems worked well internally, while failing externally. Processes were efficient, decisions were defensible, metrics looked acceptable, and yet people felt lost. They didn't know what was happening next, they didn't understand why a decision was made, and they didn't feel seen in the process. None of those failures appeared as errors, but each one eroded trust.

When trust erodes, quality weakens, even if everything is technically correct.

Patients and members do not experience healthcare as workflows. They experience it as moments. Moments of vulnerability, moments of confusion, moments of relief or frustration. Patient-centeredness asks whether systems honor those moments or ignore them in favor of internal convenience.

I have seen situations where care was clinically appropriate and timely, yet still felt unsafe because the person receiving it did not understand what was happening. Uncertainty creates fear, and fear changes behavior. People hesitate to ask questions. They delay decisions. They disengage quietly. From a quality perspective, that disengagement is a risk.

Research consistently supports this reality. Studies show that when patients feel unheard or confused, adherence drops, outcomes worsen, and utilization patterns change. These are often framed as behavioral issues, but they are design issues at their core. Systems that assume understanding create barriers for those who need clarity the most.

Patient-centeredness is where quality meets humility.

One of the biggest misconceptions I had to unlearn was the idea that patient-centeredness is subjective and therefore difficult to operationalize. In practice, it is deeply structural. It shows up in how information is presented, how choices are framed, how much effort is required to navigate care, and how predictable outcomes feel.

When systems require people to decipher complex logic during moments of stress, patient-centeredness has already failed. Quality does not improve when people must work harder to receive care. It improves when systems shoulder that burden instead.

Healthcare technology has both helped and hindered patient-centeredness. Digital tools have increased access to information and expanded touchpoints, but they have also increased complexity. Portals, notifications, automated messages, and decision pathways can overwhelm as easily as they can empower.

I have seen systems deliver accurate information at the wrong moment, in the wrong format, without context. From a technical standpoint, communication occurred. From a human standpoint, understanding did not. Patient-centeredness is not about delivering information. It is about ensuring comprehension.

This is where quality tools quietly influence patient-centeredness, even when they are not labeled as such. Journey mapping, usability testing, experience surveys, and feedback loops are often treated as secondary to clinical or operational priorities. But the organizations that use these tools well uncover friction that metrics never reveal.

When quality teams observe where people hesitate, repeat questions, or abandon processes, they gain insight into how systems feel, not just how they function. Those insights are invaluable because experience predicts behavior far better than instructions ever will.

Patient-centeredness also forces us to confront assumptions about capability. Healthcare systems often assume digital access, health literacy, time flexibility, and emotional bandwidth. Many people do not have these consistently, especially when they are sick. When systems require ideal conditions to function well, they privilege some and exclude others.

This is where patient-centeredness intersects with equity. Designing for the average user almost always leaves someone behind. Quality professionals must learn to ask who struggles most with our designs, and why. That question is uncomfortable, but it is essential.

As healthcare increasingly explores personalization through artificial intelligence, patient-centeredness faces both promise and risk. AI can tailor information, predict needs, and adjust pathways dynamically. But personalization without transparency can feel intrusive or confusing. Systems that adapt silently can undermine trust if people do not understand why outcomes change.

The future of patient-centeredness will depend on whether technology enhances understanding or replaces it. AI should help systems meet people where they are, not push people further away.

What I have come to believe is that patient-centeredness is not about anticipating every preference. It is about respecting human limits and designing accordingly. It is about recognizing that clarity is a form of care, predictability is a form of safety, and dignity is a quality outcome.

Patient-centeredness proves, perhaps more clearly than any other dimension, that quality is a mindset. It cannot be delegated to scripts or training alone. It lives in how decisions are framed, how systems respond to uncertainty, and how seriously organizations take the lived experience of those they serve.

When patient-centeredness is treated as a skillset, it becomes performative. When it is treated as a mindset, it becomes structural.

And, when systems are designed with that mindset, people don't just receive care—they feel supported by it. That feeling changes behavior. It builds trust. And it turns quality from an abstract goal into a lived reality.

Mindset in Action - Patient-Centeredness

Patient-centeredness is often approached as a communication skill. Say the right words, show empathy, and improve satisfaction scores. From a skillset perspective, success is measured by how well interactions are managed.

But patient-centeredness is not proven in conversations alone.

It is proven how systems behave when people are stressed, confused, or vulnerable.

A mindset-driven view of patient-centeredness asks whether care was understandable, predictable, and respectful, not just whether it was delivered. It recognizes that people navigating healthcare are rarely operating at full capacity. Illness, fear, financial pressure, and uncertainty narrow attention and patience. Systems that require extra effort during these moments quietly push people away.

In one healthcare workflow, instructions were accurate and complete, yet people repeatedly failed to complete the process. Rather than assuming disengagement, quality teams observed the journey step by step. They realized the system expected people to connect information across multiple messages, platforms, and timeframes. Once the pathway was simplified and explanations were sequenced to match how people actually process information, engagement improved dramatically.

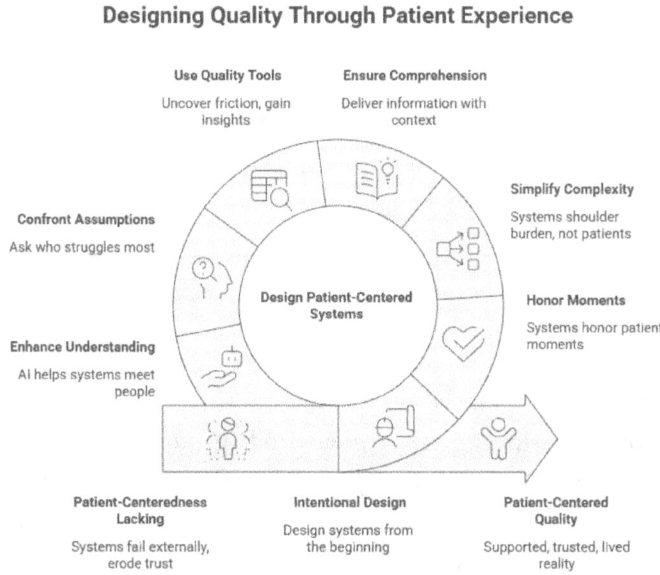

When quality is treated as a skillset, patient-centeredness becomes performance.

When quality is treated as a mindset, patient-centeredness becomes design.

And design is where experience and dignity are protected.

CHAPTER 6

Timeliness: When Time Becomes a Clinical Variable

Time behaves differently in healthcare than it does anywhere else. Inside organizations, time is measured in queues, service levels, and turnaround targets. Outside those systems, time is felt as waiting, uncertainty, and fear. I learned early on that this difference—between measured time and experienced time—is where many quality failures quietly begin.

For a long time, timeliness was explained to me as an efficiency problem. Reduce delays, improve cycle time, meet SLAs. Those goals are important, but they miss the deeper truth. In healthcare, time is not neutral. It carries emotional weight, clinical consequences, and behavioral impact. A delay does not simply slow care—it reshapes decisions.

I have seen situations where a delay was technically acceptable and still harmful. Internally, everything stayed within defined thresholds. Externally, people waited without clarity. Anxiety grew, confidence faded. Some disengaged altogether. By the time care finally arrived, the waiting itself had already compromised its effectiveness.

Timeliness is not just about speed; it is about certainty.

In the United States, access delays are widespread and consequential. Research consistently shows that a significant percentage of patients experience delays in receiving care, whether due to administrative processes, scheduling constraints, or coordination gaps. Studies estimate that **nearly one in four adults has delayed or avoided care** at some point because of system-related barriers. These delays are often discussed as utilization issues, but from a quality perspective, they are safety and effectiveness issues in disguise.

When people wait too long, conditions worsen. When uncertainty stretches, stress rises. When outcomes feel unpredictable, behavior changes, none of this is captured fully by turnaround metrics.

What changed my approach to timeliness was realizing that people don't experience delays as numbers; they experience them as silence. Silence between steps, silence after requests, silence while trying to understand what comes next. That silence is interpreted as indifference, even when no one intends it that way.

Timeliness, then, is as much about communication as it is about processing speed.

I have seen healthcare systems improve timeliness dramatically, not by accelerating everything, but by clarifying expectations. When people know what will happen next, when it will happen, and what to do in the meantime, waiting becomes tolerable. When they don't, even short delays feel unbearable.

Quality professionals often underestimate the power of predictability.

Timeliness breaks most often at transitions: hand-offs between teams, movement between systems and responsibility shifts. Each transition introduces the possibility of delay, not because anyone is careless, but because no one fully owns the time between steps. Inside organizations, these gaps feel small. To someone waiting, they feel endless.

I have learned to pay close attention to those in-between spaces. That is where timeliness quietly fails.

Technology has reshaped timeliness in complex ways. Automation has made certain decisions faster, but it has also introduced new forms of waiting. People now wait for system updates, automated determinations, or backend processes they cannot see or influence. Speed increased in one part of the system, while opacity increased in another.

From a quality perspective, faster processing does not automatically translate to better timeliness. If people cannot see progress or understand delays, speed loses its meaning.

As healthcare systems rely more heavily on digital workflows, timeliness becomes increasingly dependent on design. Systems that batch work, prioritize volume, or optimize internal efficiency can unintentionally extend waiting for those on the outside. Quality thinking must surface these trade-offs early, before delays become normalized.

The most effective approaches to timeliness I have seen treat time as a shared responsibility. They look beyond averages and focus on variability. They ask who waits the longest and why. They examine how delays affect different populations differently. They recognize that timeliness failures rarely appear as single events; they appear as patterns.

Patterns tell stories that metrics alone cannot.

Artificial intelligence is beginning to influence timeliness in new ways. Predictive models can anticipate demand, optimize scheduling, and flag cases at risk of delay. Used well, these tools can shorten wait times and improve flow. Used poorly, they can reinforce existing inequities or prioritize efficiency over urgency.

AI does not understand anxiety. It understands probability. Quality professionals must ensure that human judgment remains part of how timeliness decisions are made, especially when delays carry clinical or emotional risk.

What timeliness has taught me is that quality is not always about moving faster. Sometimes, it is about slowing down long enough to explain, to set expectations, to acknowledge uncertainty. Those moments often matter more than shaving minutes off a process.

Timeliness proves that quality is not a mechanical outcome. It is a lived experience. It is shaped by how systems handle waiting, how they communicate during uncertainty, and how they respect the fact that time feels different when health is on the line.

When timeliness is treated as a skillset, the focus stays on metrics. When it is treated as a mindset, the focus shifts to impact. That shift changes how systems are designed and how people experience care.

In healthcare, time is never just time.
It is trust measured in moments.

And quality lives in how we choose to honor it.

Mindset in Action – Timeliness

Clocks and queues often measure timeliness. Turnaround times are tracked, and service levels are met. From an internal perspective, time appears controlled and predictable.

But from the outside, time feels very different.

A mindset-driven view of timeliness recognizes that waiting is not space. It is filled with uncertainty, anxiety, and interpretation. When people wait without understanding what is happening or when it will end, trust erodes, even if timelines are technically acceptable.

In one healthcare system, internal processing times consistently met targets, yet frustration continued to rise. Quality teams discovered that the issue was not speed, but silence. Members were waiting without clarity. Once expectations were clearly communicated—what was happening, why it was taking time, and when to expect an update—engagement improved immediately, without any change in processing speed.

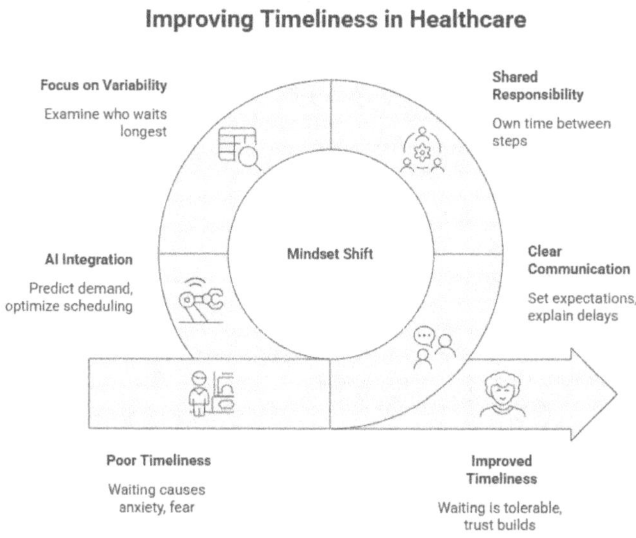

Nothing became faster.

But everything became more bearable.

When quality is treated as a skillset, timeliness is optimized inside the system.

When quality is treated as a mindset, timeliness is experienced by the person waiting.

That shift turns time from a metric into a responsibility.

CHAPTER 7

Efficiency: Removing Waste Without Removing Care

For a long time, efficiency in healthcare made me uneasy. It was often discussed in the language of cost, speed, and reduction. Reduce spend, reduce touchpoints, reduce time. On the surface, these goals made sense. Healthcare is expensive, complex, and under constant pressure to do more with less. But the more I worked in healthcare quality, the more I realized that efficiency, when misunderstood, can quietly erode the very outcomes it claims to protect.

Efficiency is not about doing less for people. It is about doing less *to* people.

What changed my thinking was recognizing how often inefficiency shows up not as inconvenience, but as harm. Rework forces people to repeat their stories. Redundant steps delay care. Escalations create anxiety. Hand-offs multiply confusion. None of these are neutral experiences. Each one consumes time, energy, and trust, resources that people seeking care often do not have to spare.

In the United States, estimates suggest that **25–30% of healthcare spending** is tied to administrative complexity and waste. That number is staggering, but it becomes even more concerning when you consider how that waste is experienced. It shows up as long calls, repeated forms, unclear next steps, and systems that ask people to navigate complexity during moments of vulnerability. From a quality perspective, inefficiency is not just a financial issue. It is an experience issue.

I have seen inefficiency blamed on individuals more times than I can count. People are told to work faster, document better, or follow processes more closely. But inefficiency rarely originates with people. It originates with design. When workflows are fragmented, when systems don't talk to each other, when rules require exceptions to function, people compensate. They build workarounds. They create shadow processes. They absorb friction so the system can keep moving.

That compensation comes at a cost.

What I have learned is that inefficiency is often the system's way of asking for help. It signals that something was designed without fully understanding how work actually happens. Quality professionals are uniquely positioned to see this because we sit close enough to outcomes to notice patterns, and far enough from day-to-day execution to question assumptions.

Efficiency improves not when people work harder, but when systems work better.

One of the most damaging myths in healthcare is that efficiency and quality conflict. I have heard it framed as a trade-off: either we move fast, or we protect people. That framing is false. Poorly designed efficiency creates risk. Thoughtful efficiency reduces it. When unnecessary steps are removed, clarity improves. When duplication is eliminated, delays shrink. When hand-offs are simplified, errors decrease.

The key difference is intention.

I have seen organizations pursue efficiency by cutting steps without understanding why those steps existed. The result was faster processes that created more confusion and more downstream work. I have also seen organizations invest time upfront to understand where effort was being wasted and redesign accordingly. Those changes didn't just reduce cost—they improved access, timeliness, and trust simultaneously.

Efficiency done well strengthens every other quality dimension.

Quality tools often enter efficiency conversations through process mapping, waste analysis, and continuous improvement initiatives. These tools are powerful when used to understand reality, not enforce ideology. When teams map workflows honestly, including workarounds, delays, and rework, they uncover truths that metrics alone never reveal.

The most valuable efficiency insights I have seen have come from listening to the people doing the work and the people experiencing it. Where do things slow down? Where do questions repeat? Where does effort multiply without adding value? Those questions reveal where quality thinking needs to be applied, not where people need to be pushed harder.

Technology has dramatically reshaped efficiency in healthcare. Automation has eliminated manual steps, accelerated decisions, and scaled processes. In many ways, it has delivered exactly what it promised. But it has also exposed a new risk: automating inefficiency simply allows waste to happen faster.

I have seen systems that executed inefficient logic flawlessly. The result was consistency, not improvement. Quality professionals must be involved before automation occurs, asking whether what is being automated actually makes sense. Efficiency cannot be achieved by speeding up a flawed process. It must be redesigned at the source.

As artificial intelligence becomes more integrated into healthcare workflows, efficiency will be reframed. AI can reduce administrative burden, predict needs, and streamline decision-making. Used thoughtfully, it can return time to both caregivers and patients. Used carelessly, it can obscure accountability and amplify complexity behind the scenes.

Efficiency in the future will depend on transparency as much as speed.

What efficiency has taught me most clearly is that quality is revealed in how systems respect people's time. Every unnecessary step sends a message. Every repeated explanation erodes trust. Every avoidable delay changes behavior. Efficiency is not about squeezing more output from systems. It is about removing friction that never should have existed in the first place.

When efficiency is treated as a skillset, it becomes a cost-cutting exercise. When it is treated as a mindset, it becomes an act of care.

Quality professionals who approach efficiency with that mindset ask different questions. They ask whose effort is being wasted, they ask which steps exist out of habit rather than purpose, they ask how to simplify without oversimplifying, and how to remove burden without removing support.

Efficiency is not the absence of work.

It is the presence of intention.

And, when efficiency is designed with that intention, healthcare becomes not only more sustainable, but more humane.

Mindset in Action – Efficiency

Efficiency in healthcare is often pursued with intensity. Reduce costs, remove steps, automate decisions. From a skillset perspective, efficiency is about streamlining and output.

But efficiency that ignores experience relocates waste, instead of removing it.

A mindset-driven approach to efficiency looks for friction before it looks for cuts. It pays attention to repeated questions, workarounds, escalations, and rework, not as failures of people, but as signals of poor design. It recognizes that when systems rely on human compensation to function, inefficiency is already embedded.

In one automated workflow, processing time dropped significantly after a manual review step was removed. On paper, efficiency improved. In reality, exception cases increased, escalations multiplied, and both staff and members absorbed more effort. When quality teams redesigned the logic to anticipate variability rather than optimize for the average case, overall effort declined across the system.

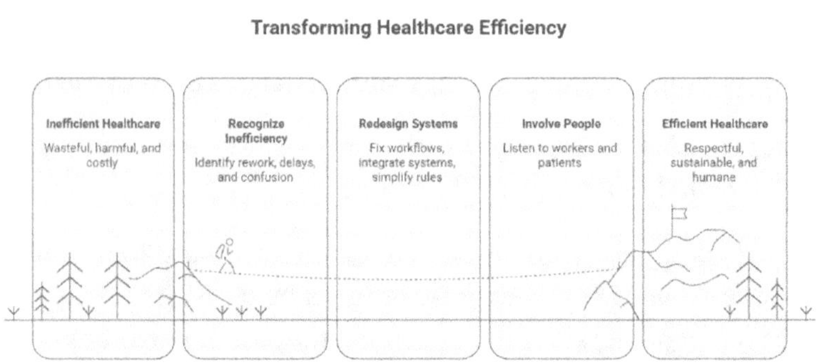

Efficiency improved, not by doing less work, but by removing work that never should have existed.

When quality is treated as a skillset, efficiency becomes a cost exercise.

When quality is treated as a mindset, efficiency becomes an act of respect for people's time and energy.

That is what makes efficiency sustainable.

Moment That Changed My Thinking: Faster Was Not Better

We once redesigned a workflow to improve turnaround time. A manual review step was removed, and automation handled it perfectly. Processing time improved significantly, and leadership celebrated.

A month later, exceptional cases increased. Escalations multiplied. Staff were working harder than before, just in different places.

We had optimized speed, but we hadn't redesigned the logic. We had accelerated it.

I remember thinking:

We didn't remove work.

We relocated it.

We reintroduced judgment earlier in the process. We redesigned the logic to account for variability, instead of average cases.

Efficiency improved—not because we cut steps, but because we removed friction that never should have existed.

That was the day I understood:

Efficiency without empathy becomes a burden.

CHAPTER 8

Equity: When Quality Works for Everyone, Not Just the Average

For a long time, equity felt like something discussed on the edges of healthcare quality—important, aspirational, but somehow separate from the core work. Safety, effectiveness, timeliness, and efficiency were treated as operational priorities. Equity was treated as a value statement. That separation never sat well with me, but it took years of experience to understand why.

Equity is not an add-on to quality. It is the test of whether quality actually exists.

I began to see this clearly when I noticed a pattern that repeated itself across systems and settings. The same process would work beautifully for some people and fail quietly for others. The metrics looked acceptable. The averages told a reassuring story. But the lived experiences underneath those averages were very different. Some people moved through care smoothly. Others struggled, stalled, or disengaged, not because they were unwilling, but because the system assumed conditions they did not have.

That is where equity reveals itself.

In the United States, disparities in healthcare access and outcomes are well-documented. Differences in income, geography, race, language, and education consistently correlate with differences in health outcomes. These disparities are often discussed as social problems, but from a quality perspective, they are design problems. Systems that work only when people have time, resources, literacy, and flexibility are systems designed for a narrow slice of reality.

Quality, which depends on privilege, is not quality.

I have seen how seemingly neutral decisions create inequitable outcomes. A process that requires frequent follow-up favors those who can take time off work. Digital-first pathways favor those with reliable access and comfort with technology. Complex instructions favor those with high health literacy. None of these decisions is malicious. Most are made for efficiency or standardization. But their impact is uneven, and that unevenness accumulates into disparity.

Equity forces quality professionals to ask not just whether a system works, but *for whom* it works.

One of the most challenging aspects of equity is that it is often invisible to those who benefit from existing designs. When systems work smoothly for us, it is easy to assume they work smoothly for everyone. Equity work begins when we question that assumption and seek out voices that are not represented in our metrics.

Experience data, when collected and interpreted thoughtfully, can surface these gaps. But equity is not revealed by satisfaction scores alone. It shows up in who disengages, who delays care, and who never completes a journey. It shows up in patterns of silence as much as in complaints.

Listening for absence is one of the most important equity practices I have learned.

Healthcare quality tools are increasingly being used to examine disparities, stratifying outcomes, identifying gaps, and measuring variation across populations. These tools are valuable, but they are not enough on their own. Data can tell us where inequities exist, but it cannot tell us why unless we are willing to look beyond numbers.

I have seen equity initiatives fail because they focused on reporting disparities rather than redesigning systems. Awareness is necessary, but action requires humility. It requires acknowledging that systems built for efficiency or scale may need to change to serve people more fairly.

Equity often challenges comfort.

Technology has both exposed and amplified equity challenges. Digital health tools have expanded access for many, but they have also widened gaps for those without connectivity, language support, or digital literacy.

Automated systems can unintentionally reinforce bias if they are trained on incomplete or skewed data. AI, in particular, reflects the assumptions embedded in its design.

The future of equity in healthcare will depend on who is included in design decisions and whose data shapes predictions. AI can be a powerful force for equity, identifying underserved populations, predicting barriers, and personalizing support. But without intentional oversight, it can just as easily codify inequity at scale.

Equity requires vigilance, not just innovation.

What equity has taught me is that quality is not proven by excellence at the center. It is proven by consistency at the edges. Systems that truly deliver quality do not ask people to adapt to complexity. They adapt complexity to people.

That adaptation requires a mindset shift. It requires moving away from designing for the average and toward designing for variability. It requires recognizing that fairness does not mean sameness. It means responsiveness.

When equity is treated as a skillset, it becomes a compliance exercise—policies, statements, initiatives. When it is treated as a mindset, it becomes a design principle. Decisions are made differently. Trade-offs are evaluated through a broader lens. Success is defined not only by overall improvement but by whether gaps are closing.

Equity ultimately reveals the heart of healthcare quality. It asks whether we are willing to see the people our systems struggle to serve, and whether we are willing to change because of what we see.

Quality is not a mindset when it works only for some.
It becomes a mindset when it works for everyone.
And equity is how we know the difference.

Mindset in Action – Equity

Equity is often addressed through measurement. Outcomes are stratified, gaps are identified, and differences are acknowledged. From a skillset perspective, progress feels tangible once disparities are documented.

But equity is not resolved by awareness alone.

A mindset-driven approach to equity asks who struggles with systems that appear to work well. It looks beyond averages and into lived experience. It pays attention to who disengages, who delays care, and who never makes it far enough to appear in the data.

In one healthcare initiative, digital access expanded and overall performance metrics improved. Yet, certain populations participated less over time. When quality teams examined the design assumptions, they found that the pathway required stable connectivity, digital literacy, and flexibility that not everyone had. By redesigning entry points and support options, access improved for those previously excluded—without diminishing outcomes for anyone else.

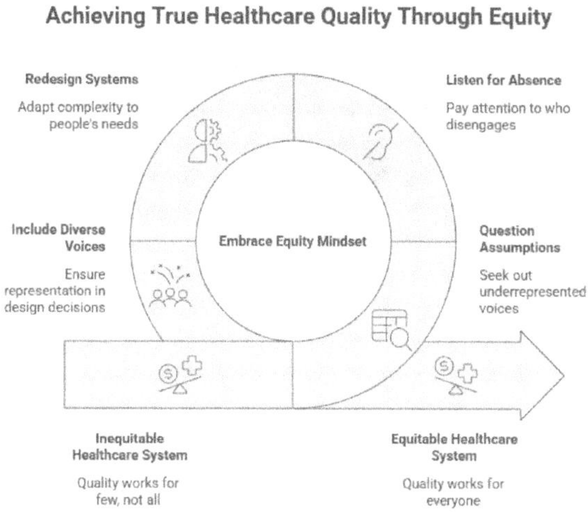
Achieving True Healthcare Quality Through Equity
Redesign Systems
Adapt complexity to people's needs
Listen for Absence
Pay attention to who disengages
Include Diverse Voices
Ensure representation in design decisions
Embrace Equity Mindset
Question Assumptions
Seek out underrepresented voices
Inequitable Healthcare System
Quality works for few, not all
Equitable Healthcare System
Quality works for everyone

Equity did not require new intent.
It required new humility.

When quality is treated as a skillset, equity becomes a reporting obligation.

When quality is treated as a mindset, equity becomes a design responsibility.

And that responsibility determines whether healthcare quality truly serves everyone, or only those it was unconsciously built for.

CHAPTER 9

How Quality Decisions Ripple: What Happens After We Say "Yes"

One of the most difficult lessons I learned in healthcare quality is that the most important quality decisions often don't feel important at the time they are made. They happen quietly, in meetings that move too fast, in assumptions that seem reasonable, and in moments when the pressure to proceed outweighs the urge to pause. By the time a member experiences the impact, the decision is long past, documented, approved and forgotten.

Quality rarely breaks where it is noticed. It breaks where it was never fully considered.

I used to think that quality failures showed up as obvious errors—something incorrect, something misconfigured, something broken. Over time, I realized that many quality failures come from decisions that were technically correct but contextually incomplete. The system worked. The logic fired. The process followed its path. And yet, the outcome felt wrong to the person experiencing it.

This is where the idea of "ripple effects" became real for me.

Every decision in healthcare creates movement. A clarification here, a rule there, a timing change somewhere else. None of these exists in isolation. They interact with real people, real schedules, real stress, and real constraints. When we evaluate quality only at the point of execution, we miss how those interactions compound.

I have seen this play out repeatedly. A change is reviewed and approved because it meets documented requirements. Testing passes because scenarios were designed around expected behavior. Operational readiness is confirmed because all stakeholders signed off. From the inside, the change looks successful. From the outside, access slows down, confusion increases, or costs become unpredictable. Nothing "failed" in the traditional sense. But quality still suffered.

What I have learned is that healthcare quality does not fail because systems malfunction. It fails because **systems behave exactly as designed in environments that were never fully imagined**.

Healthcare IT plays a powerful role in this dynamic. Modern systems are capable of executing decisions at an extraordinary scale. They are consistent, fast and relentless. Once logic is implemented, it doesn't pause to ask whether the context has shifted or whether the person on the other end understands what just happened. It simply executes.

That scale is both an advantage and a risk.

A single design assumption, when automated, can affect thousands or millions of people. A small timing dependency can cascade into widespread delays. A narrow interpretation of policy can quietly restrict access in ways that no one intended. The system does not see harm. It only sees logic.

This is where quality professionals become essential, not as validators of correctness, but as anticipators of consequence.

I have noticed that the most fragile points in healthcare quality are not within individual tasks, but at the boundaries. Where one team hands off to another, where policy is translated into system behavior, where timing overlaps, where responsibility becomes shared, and therefore diluted, these boundary zones are where assumptions hide and where ripple effects begin.

Research consistently shows that a large percentage of healthcare issues—some estimates place it above **60%**—are tied not to isolated failures, but to communication gaps, hand-offs, and coordination breakdowns. These are not skill problems; they are system problems. Systems problems require quality professionals who are willing to think beyond their immediate scope.

One of the most challenging shifts for me was learning to evaluate quality decisions not by whether they passed review, but by how they would behave once they left the controlled environment of planning and entered the unpredictability of real life. How would this decision feel to someone already anxious about their health? What happens if their situation doesn't fit the standard scenario? What if timing matters more than logic? What if cost changes behavior?

These questions are not always comfortable, especially when timelines are tight and confidence is high. But I have learned that discomfort at the decision stage is far less costly than distress at the point of care.

There is a common belief in healthcare that issues can be fixed later, and sometimes they can. But quality work teaches you that later is often too late. By the time an issue surfaces visibly, trust has already been damaged, behavior has already changed, and safety may already be compromised. Prevention is quieter, but far more powerful.

"Quality is not about fixing what breaks.
It is about noticing what might break before it does."

I have also learned that many ripple effects don't look dramatic. They show up as small increases in call volume, longer resolution times, repeated explanations, or subtle frustration. But these small signals matter. Over time, they accumulate into dissatisfaction, disengagement, and avoidance. In healthcare, avoidance is dangerous.

Studies show that when patients experience confusion or unexpected barriers, adherence drops significantly—sometimes by **15–25%**. That drop is rarely attributed to quality design, but it should be. People don't disengage because they don't care. They disengage because the system made care harder than it needed to be.

Quality professionals sit in a unique position. We are close enough to decisions to influence them, but far enough from the point of care to forget their human impact if we're not intentional. This chapter is a reminder that quality work does not end at approval. It begins there.

As healthcare continues to evolve with more automation, faster deployments, and increasing reliance on data-driven decisions, the ripple effects of quality thinking will only grow. The future will reward those who can slow down at the right moments, ask deeper questions, and see beyond immediate success indicators.

Before moving on, I invite you to pause again. Think about the decisions you've been part of recently. Which ones felt small at the time but had a wide impact later? Where did assumptions go unchallenged? Where did "good enough" quietly replace "safe and clear"?

Those reflections are not about regret. They are about growth.

Because once you begin to see how quality decisions ripple, you can no longer unsee it. And when you can't unsee it, your role in healthcare quality changes permanently.

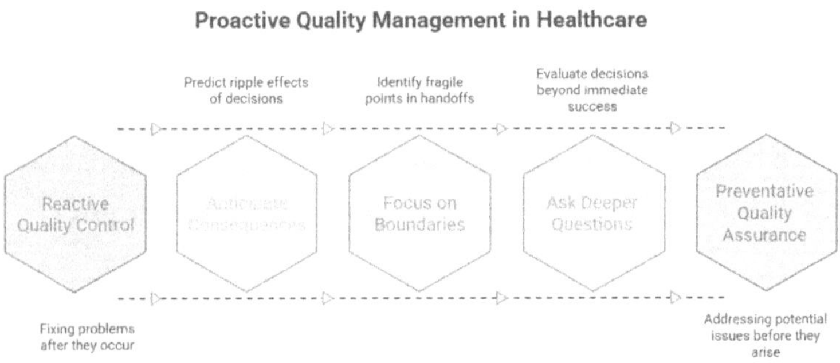
Proactive Quality Management in Healthcare
Predict ripple effects of decisions
Identify fragile points in handoffs
Evaluate decisions beyond immediate success
Reactive Quality Control
Focus on Boundaries
Ask Deeper Questions
Preventative Quality Assurance
Fixing problems after they occur
Addressing potential issues before they arise

CHAPTER 10

Access to Care: Where Quality Becomes Real

There is a moment in every healthcare journey when quality stops being theoretical and becomes personal. It is the moment someone tries to access care. Not when a policy is written, not when a system is configured, not when a metric is reported, but when a real person needs help and reaches out to the system, expecting a response.

That moment is where quality either shows up or quietly disappears.

Over the years, I have come to believe that access to care is the most honest measure of healthcare quality. You can have strong policies, advanced technology and impressive dashboards, but if someone cannot get the care they need at the time they need it, quality has already failed. Everything else becomes a justification after the fact.

Access is often treated as an operational issue. Backlogs, queues, capacity constraints, and scheduling challenges. Those are real concerns, but they are not the full story. From a quality perspective, access is the outcome of dozens of upstream decisions, many of which happen far away from the person trying to get care. When access breaks down, it is rarely because someone decided to block care. It is because quality thinking stopped too early.

I have seen this play out in subtle ways. A rule that was meant to standardize decisions introduces an extra step that no one anticipated. A timing dependency creates a gap between when care is needed and when the system is ready to respond. A clarification meant to improve consistency adds ambiguity for those navigating the system for the first time. None of these are malicious decisions. But their impact is very real.

From the inside, access looks like eligibility checks, approvals, workflows and system logic. From the outside, access feels like waiting, uncertainty and sometimes helplessness. That difference in perspective matters more than we often acknowledge.

One of the hardest things to accept in healthcare quality is that **access delayed is often access denied**, at least temporarily. And temporary denial can still cause harm. A delay can worsen a condition, increase anxiety, force people to make choices they wouldn't otherwise make, and in some cases, push people away from the system entirely.

Research consistently shows that when access is complicated or delayed, people disengage. Studies estimate that nearly **one in five patients delay or avoid care** due to barriers related to access, clarity, or cost. These are not fringe cases; they are everyday experiences for millions of people.

What makes access such a powerful quality indicator is that it reflects multiple dimensions at once. Safety, timeliness, effectiveness, equity, and trust all converge at the point of access. When access works well, people feel supported, even when outcomes are uncertain. When it doesn't, frustration and fear fill the gap.

I have learned that access issues rarely originate where they surface. They often begin with assumptions about how people will navigate the system. Assumptions about timing, assumptions about understanding, assumptions about resources. When those assumptions don't hold—and they often don't—the burden falls on the person seeking care.

Healthcare IT plays a significant role here. Systems are designed to apply logic consistently, which is necessary at scale. But consistency, without context, can become rigidity. A system cannot sense urgency. It cannot recognize when waiting becomes dangerous. It cannot distinguish between inconvenience and harm. That distinction must be built into design—and protected by quality judgment.

One of the most important shifts in my thinking was realizing that access is not a single gate. It is a journey. A person moves through multiple checkpoints, some visible, many invisible, before care actually happens. Each checkpoint introduces the possibility of delay, confusion or friction. Quality professionals influence many of those checkpoints, often without realizing it.

"Access is not about whether care exists.
It's about whether care can actually be reached.

The best-performing healthcare organizations I have observed treat access as a shared quality responsibility. They don't isolate it within one team or function. They look at access holistically, across systems, processes, and communication. They design pathways that anticipate real-world behavior rather than ideal scenarios. They monitor early signals, not just outcomes.

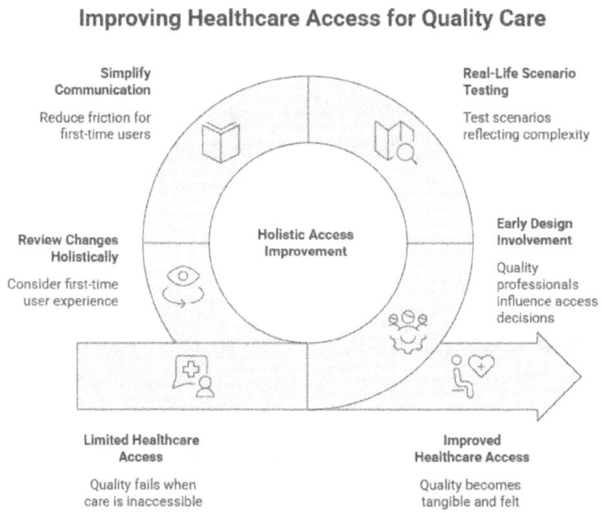
Improving Healthcare Access for Quality Care
Simplify Communication
Reduce friction for first-time users
Real-Life Scenario Testing
Test scenarios reflecting complexity
Holistic Access Improvement
Review Changes Holistically
Consider first-time user experience
Early Design Involvement
Quality professionals influence access decisions
Limited Healthcare Access
Quality fails when care is inaccessible
Improved Healthcare Access
Quality becomes tangible and felt

Some best practices that consistently make a difference include involving quality professionals early in access-related design decisions, testing scenarios that reflect real-life complexity, simplifying communication wherever possible, and reviewing changes through the lens of how a first-time user would experience them. These practices don't eliminate all access challenges, but they significantly reduce avoidable friction.

The future of healthcare will place even greater pressure on access. As systems become faster and more automated, the margin for misunderstanding shrinks. Decisions will be made in seconds, but their impact may last much longer. In that environment, quality professionals must become even more vigilant about how access pathways behave under real conditions.

Access to care is where healthcare promises are tested. It is where quality becomes tangible. It is also where failures are felt most deeply.

As you read this chapter, I encourage you to think about access not as someone else's problem, but as a direct outcome of quality thinking. Ask yourself where your decisions might influence access, even indirectly. Ask where assumptions might be adding friction. Ask what it feels like to experience the system from the outside.

Those questions don't slow progress; they protect it.

Because when access works, quality feels invisible.

And when it doesn't, nothing else matters.

Mindset in Action – Access to Care

Access is often defined by eligibility, availability, and network inclusion. From a skillset perspective, access exists if care is technically offered and rules are followed.

But access that cannot be navigated is access in name only.

A mindset-driven approach to access recognizes that the journey to care matters as much as the endpoint. It asks whether people can realistically move through each step without confusion, delay, or financial fear. It treats friction not as an inconvenience but as a barrier that changes behavior.

In one system, access rules were applied correctly and consistently. Yet, utilization dropped among certain groups. Quality teams discovered that while care was technically available, the steps required to reach it were unclear and intimidating. By clarifying entry points, setting expectations, and reducing unnecessary hand-offs, access improved—without changing coverage or eligibility at all.

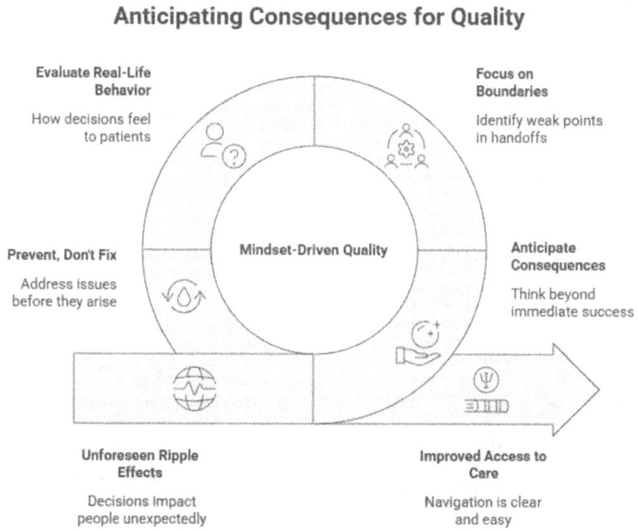
Anticipating Consequences for Quality
Evaluate Real-Life Behavior
How decisions feel to patients
Focus on Boundaries
Identify weak points in handoffs
Mindset-Driven Quality
Prevent, Don't Fix
Address issues before they arise
Anticipate Consequences
Think beyond immediate success
Unforeseen Ripple Effects
Decisions impact people unexpectedly
Improved Access to Care
Navigation is clear and easy

Access expanded not because rules changed, but because navigation improved.

When quality is treated as a skillset, access is confirmed at approval.

When quality is treated as a mindset, access is confirmed on arrival.

That distinction determines whether care is reachable or merely promised

CHAPTER 11

When Cost Becomes Risk: Why Financial Impact Is Patient Safety

For a long time in healthcare, we separated financial conversations from safety conversations. Cost lived in one room. Clinical risk lived in another. Quality sat somewhere in between, trying to translate both. Over the years, I have come to believe that this separation is one of the quietest and most dangerous mistakes we make.

When people cannot afford care, safety is already compromised.

I didn't fully understand this early in my career. Like many quality professionals, I viewed financial outcomes as downstream effects, important but not central to safety. That perspective changed as I began to see patterns. People are delaying care because of cost, people are skipping doses to make prescriptions last longer, and people are abandoning treatment plans altogether because the financial burden feels unpredictable or overwhelming. None of these behaviors showed up as clinical errors, but all of them increased risk.

Financial stress changes behavior, and behavior is a patient safety variable.

Healthcare systems often assume rational decision-making. But illness, uncertainty and cost anxiety do not create rational conditions. They create fear. When someone is forced to choose between paying for care and meeting basic needs, the system has already placed them in an unsafe position.

Research consistently supports this. Studies estimate that nearly **40% of adults in the United States struggle to afford healthcare expenses**, and a significant portion report delaying or avoiding care due to cost concerns. Among patients managing chronic conditions, cost-related non-adherence rates range from **20–30%**. These are not marginal numbers. They represent millions of people navigating unsafe trade-offs created by financial pressure.

From a quality perspective, the most troubling part is that financial harm is often invisible until it becomes severe. Unlike clinical events, financial distress doesn't always trigger immediate alarms. It accumulates quietly. Bills arrive later, confusion lingers, stress compounds. By the time the impact surfaces, trust has already eroded.

Quality professionals influence this more than we often realize.

Even when we are not setting prices or designing benefits, we shape the financial experience through decisions about clarity, predictability and system behavior. We influence how rules are interpreted, how exceptions are handled, how changes are communicated and how edge cases are treated. Each of these choices can either protect people from financial shock or expose them to it.

I have seen situations where systems behaved exactly as designed, yet cost changes blindsided people they did not understand or anticipate. From the inside, everything looked compliant. From the outside, it felt unfair. That disconnect matters because fairness is a cornerstone of trust.

One of the most difficult truths to accept in healthcare quality is that **correctness does not guarantee safety**. A decision can align perfectly with policy and still produce harm if it creates financial barriers that alter health behavior. When people begin rationing care, delaying treatment, or disengaging from the system altogether, the risk shifts from theoretical to real.

"If a system forces people to choose between health and affordability, the system is unsafe."

Financial impact also intersects deeply with equity. Cost burdens do not affect everyone equally. They weigh more heavily on people with limited resources, chronic conditions, or less flexibility in their lives. When systems assume that people can absorb unexpected costs or navigate complex explanations, they unintentionally widen disparities. Quality work must acknowledge this reality.

Healthcare IT plays a significant role in shaping financial experiences. Automated systems apply rules consistently, but consistency does not always feel fair. Without thoughtful design and clear communication, automation can amplify financial harm at scale. A small configuration decision can affect thousands of people overnight. Quality professionals act as the human lens that asks, "What will this feel like when it reaches real life?"

The most effective organizations I have observed treat financial transparency as a quality outcome. They prioritize clarity over complexity. They test scenarios that reflect real-world affordability challenges. They monitor early signals of confusion and distress, not just outcomes. And they involve quality professionals early when financial behavior is likely to change.

As healthcare continues to evolve, financial pressure will only increase. Costs are rising faster than wages. Coverage designs are becoming more complex. Expectations for transparency are growing. In this environment, treating financial impact as "someone else's problem" is no longer viable.

Quality professionals must expand their definition of safety to include financial harm, not because we control every cost, but because we influence how systems behave under financial stress.

As you read this chapter, I invite you to reflect on how financial outcomes show up in your work. Where might people be surprised? Where might cost change behavior? Where might clarity reduce harm before it occurs?

These questions are not about assigning blame; they are about recognizing responsibility.

Because when cost becomes a barrier to care, quality has already crossed into patient safety territory.

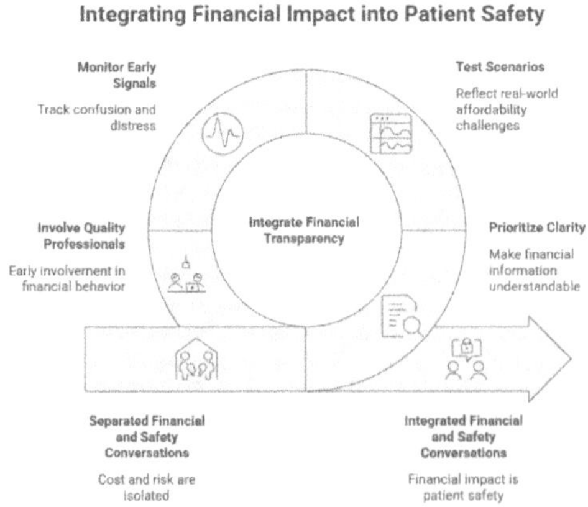
Integrating Financial Impact into Patient Safety
Monitor Early Signals
Track confusion and distress
Test Scenarios
Reflect real-world affordability challenges
Integrate Financial Transparency
Involve Quality Professionals
Early involvement in financial behavior
Prioritize Clarity
Make financial information understandable
Separated Financial and Safety Conversations
Cost and risk are isolated
Integrated Financial and Safety Conversations
Financial impact is patient safety

CHAPTER 12

Technology, Automation, AI and the Limits of Quality Without Judgment

Healthcare has always relied on tools. What has changed is the speed, scale and authority we now give those tools. Over the past decade, healthcare systems have become faster, more automated and more data-driven than ever before. Decisions that once took days now happen in seconds. Rules that once required human review are now executed automatically. From the outside, this looks like progress, and in many ways, it is.

But progress, without judgment, introduces a different kind of risk.

Early in my career, technology felt like support. Over time, it began to feel like a decision-maker. I started noticing how quickly people deferred to systems simply because they were consistent, fast, or "designed that way." The more reliable the technology appeared, the less often its assumptions were questioned. That is where quality challenges quietly began to grow.

Healthcare technology is exceptionally good at executing logic. Systems apply rules exactly as written; they scale decisions flawlessly. They do not forget steps, grow tired, or deviate from the process. These are real strengths. But systems do not understand nuance, they do not recognize distress, they do not interpret fairness, they do not ask whether an outcome *feels* reasonable to the person experiencing it.

When we forget that distinction, we begin to confuse automation with judgment.

I have seen situations where systems worked exactly as designed, yet outcomes felt deeply wrong. Access slowed, costs surprised people, and confusion increased. From a technical standpoint, nothing was broken.

From a quality standpoint, something essential was missing. The missing piece was not better code – it was better thinking.

Automation does not remove responsibility.
It concentrates it.

When a manual process fails, the impact is limited. When an automated process fails, the impact scales instantly. A small design oversight can affect thousands or millions of people before anyone notices. That reality places enormous responsibility on those involved early in design, validation, and approval. Quality professionals sit directly in that responsibility zone.

What makes this especially dangerous is the false sense of safety automation can create. When systems behave consistently, teams assume outcomes are predictable. When dashboards are green, risk feels low. But consistency does not guarantee safety, and metrics rarely capture human experience.

Research across healthcare and other high-reliability industries shows that overreliance on automation can actually *increase* risk when human oversight diminishes. Automated systems may reduce certain errors while introducing new ones—errors rooted in complacency, misunderstanding, and unchallenged assumptions. The problem is not automation itself. It is how humans relate to it.

In healthcare quality, the most concerning phrase I have heard is, "*That's just how the system works.*"

That sentence ends curiosity, it replaces judgment with acceptance, and it allows harm to persist quietly.

Quality professionals must remain skeptical, not of people, but of assumptions. Not of technology, but of completeness. Our role is not to resist automation, but to humanize it.

One of the most important questions I have learned to ask is simple: *What happens when reality doesn't match design?* Because in healthcare, reality rarely does. Appointments are missed, coverage changes mid-treatment, conditions worsen unexpectedly, and life interrupts logic. Systems that cannot adapt to these realities create friction, and friction creates risk.

Technology executes decisions.
Quality decides whether those decisions should exist.

The best healthcare organizations I have observed understand this balance. They treat technology as an enabler, not an authority. They involve quality professionals early, not after deployment. They test edge cases seriously, not as an afterthought. They ask how decisions will feel to real people, not just how they perform in controlled environments.

Artificial intelligence intensifies both the opportunity and the responsibility.

AI can identify patterns humans might miss. It can anticipate risk, predict delays, personalize outreach, and surface inequities. Used thoughtfully, it can strengthen every dimension of healthcare quality. But AI does not understand the meaning the way humans do. It recognizes patterns, not consequences. It predicts likelihood, not moral weight.

An AI model can identify who is likely to miss follow-up care, but it cannot feel the fear that causes hesitation. It can optimize schedules, but it cannot understand what waiting feels like when health is uncertain. It can flag inefficiencies, but it cannot judge whether simplification removed something essential.

AI reflects our priorities.
If those priorities are incomplete, AI will faithfully reproduce that incompleteness, at scale.

This is where the role of the quality professional must evolve. Quality can no longer be limited to auditing outcomes after the fact. We must participate earlier, in design conversations, automation decisions, and model development. We must ask how systems behave when assumptions fail, how decisions affect people who do not fit the average, and how accountability is preserved when automation obscures visibility.

The future of healthcare quality will not be defined by how advanced our tools become. It will be defined by how wisely we use them.

Healthcare systems will become more complex, not less. Care will span settings. Decisions will be shared between humans and machines. In that environment, quality will depend less on enforcing compliance and more on cultivating judgment.

Judgment cannot be automated.

That does not mean technology has limits—it means people must set them. Quality professionals must become translators between systems and humanity, ensuring that speed does not replace thought, efficiency does not replace compassion, and optimization does not replace accountability.

This chapter exists not to predict the future, but to clarify responsibility. Technology will continue to evolve. AI will become more powerful. Data will become more predictive. None of that guarantees better quality.

Quality improves only when the mindset guiding these tools is grounded in respect for human experience, awareness of unintended consequences, and the courage to pause when something feels misaligned.

The future of healthcare quality is not digital or human.
It is decisive.

Mindset in Action

Technology in healthcare is often trusted because it is consistent. Decisions are fast, and logic is applied uniformly. From a skillset perspective, success is measured by system performance and uptime.

But consistency without judgment can quietly magnify harm.

A mindset-driven approach to technology and AI recognizes that automated decisions shape human behavior, often invisibly. It asks whether people understand outcomes, whether exceptions are anticipated, and whether someone remains accountable when logic meets reality.

In one healthcare system, an automated decision pathway performed exactly as designed, yet escalations increased and trust declined. Quality teams discovered that while outcomes were technically correct, explanations were absent, and edge cases were mishandled. Once human review was reintroduced for high-impact decisions and transparency improved, outcomes stabilized, without reducing automation.

Technology did not fail.
The assumptions behind it did.

When quality is treated as a skillset, technology becomes a shortcut.

When quality is treated as a mindset, technology becomes a responsibility.

And that responsibility will define whether healthcare's future is merely faster or genuinely better.

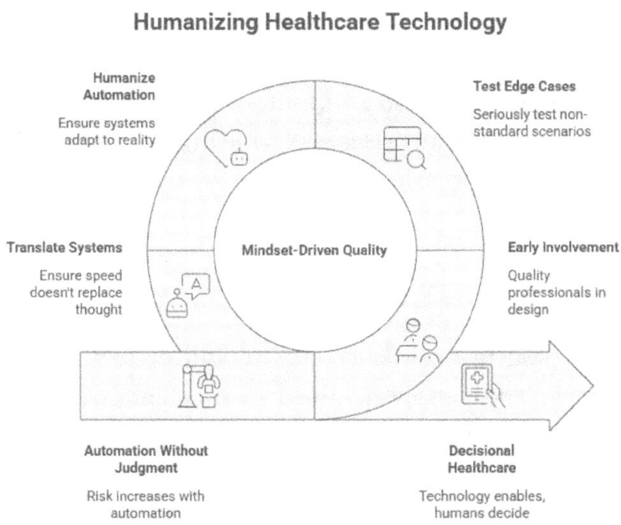

CHAPTER 13

Human Error, System Design, and Why Blame Never Improves Quality

At some point in every healthcare professional's career, something goes wrong. A decision leads to an unintended outcome. A step is missed. A handoff fails. The result surprises everyone involved. When that happens, the first instinct is often to ask, "Who made the mistake?"

I used to ask that question too.

Over time, I learned that it is almost always the wrong place to start.

The longer I worked in healthcare quality and patient safety, the more I noticed a pattern. The people involved in incidents were rarely careless, untrained, or indifferent. They were usually experienced, thoughtful, and trying to do the right thing under pressure. And yet, harm still occurred. That realization forced me to confront an uncomfortable truth: **most errors are not failures of people, but failures of systems designed without enough respect for human limits.**

Human beings are not machines. We get tired, we multitask, we make assumptions, we work with incomplete information, and we adapt when systems don't fit reality. In healthcare, we often design processes that assume perfect attention, perfect timing, and perfect understanding. When reality inevitably falls short of those assumptions, we call it human error.

But what we are really seeing is predictable behavior in imperfect systems.

I have seen organizations respond to errors by retraining individuals, issuing reminders, or tightening controls around a single step. Sometimes, those actions provide temporary reassurance. Rarely do they prevent recurrence. The same patterns resurface because the underlying conditions remain unchanged. Blame may satisfy the need for accountability, but it does very little to improve safety.

What actually improves safety is curiosity.

When quality professionals ask different questions, different insights emerge. Instead of "Who failed?" we ask, "What made this failure possible?" Instead of "Why didn't they follow the process?" we ask, "Was the process realistic?" Instead of "Why didn't someone catch this?" we ask, "What signals were missed or silenced?"

Those questions lead us away from punishment and toward design.

Research in patient safety consistently shows that a large proportion of adverse events, some studies estimate **over 70%**, are associated with communication breakdowns, handoff failures, or system complexity rather than individual negligence. These are not problems that can be solved through vigilance alone. They require structural change.

One of the most dangerous side effects of blame is silence. When people fear being held personally responsible for systemic failures, they stop speaking up. Risks go unreported, near misses are hidden, and learning slows. Over time, the organization becomes less safe, not more.

Quality professionals play a critical role in shaping how organizations respond to error. We influence whether incidents become moments of learning or moments of fear. We influence whether people feel safe raising concerns early or wait until the impact is unavoidable.

I have learned that psychological safety is not a "soft" concept. It is a safety mechanism. Teams that feel safe to admit uncertainty surface risks earlier. Teams that fear blame surface them later, or not at all. In healthcare, late awareness is often the difference between prevention and harm.

One of the most powerful shifts in my own practice was learning to see errors as signals. Signals that something in the system needs attention, signals that assumptions no longer hold, signals that complexity has outpaced design. When we treat errors this way, quality work becomes proactive rather than reactive.

"If the system requires perfection from humans, the system is unsafe."

Healthcare IT and automation add another layer to this conversation. Automated systems reduce certain types of error, but they also introduce new ones, especially when humans are expected to understand, override, or adapt to complex logic under pressure. When errors occur in automated environments, the instinct to blame individuals can be even stronger. After all, "the system told them what to do."

But systems don't tell people how to think. They tell them what to execute. When the design is unclear or the context is missing, humans are left to fill the gap. That gap is where errors often occur.

The most effective quality teams I have worked with treat error analysis as a design exercise. They map how information flowed, examine where decisions were constrained, ask what pressures were present, look for patterns rather than culprits, and focus on changes that make the right action easier and the wrong action harder.

This approach does not remove accountability. It deepens it. Accountability shifts from individuals to systems, from reactions to prevention, from hindsight to foresight.

As healthcare continues to grow more complex, the cost of ignoring human factors will only increase. Faster systems mean less time to recover from errors. Larger scale means greater impact. In this environment, quality professionals must become students of human behavior, not just system performance.

As you reflect on this chapter, think about how errors are discussed in your environment. Are they treated as failures to be hidden or opportunities to learn? Are people encouraged to raise concerns early or rewarded for staying quiet and moving fast? Do processes assume ideal behavior, or do they anticipate real human limits?

These questions matter because quality is not improved by perfection; it is improved by understanding.

And understanding begins when we stop blaming people for behaving like humans.

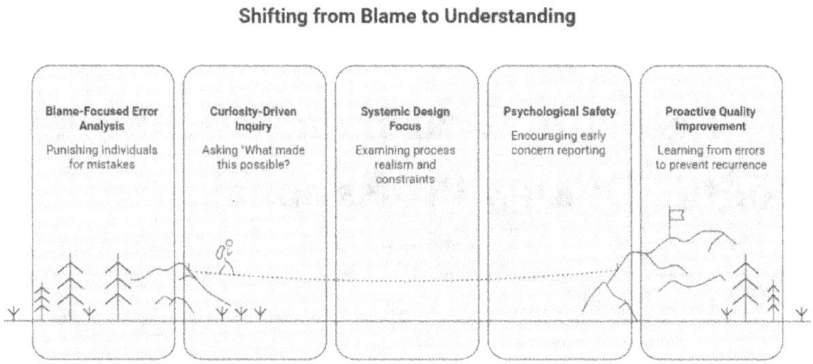
Shifting from Blame to Understanding
Blame-Focused Error Analysis
Punishing individuals for mistakes
Curiosity-Driven Inquiry
Asking "What made this possible?
Systemic Design Focus
Examining process realism and constraints
Psychological Safety
Encouraging early concern reporting
Proactive Quality Improvement
Learning from errors to prevent recurrence

CHAPTER 14

From Checker to Guardian: Redefining the Role of the Quality Professional

There was a time in my career when I believed my job in quality was to check. Check requirements, check configurations, check outputs, check boxes. I took pride in being thorough, precise, and consistent. And for a while, that felt like enough.

But over time, something started to bother me.

I noticed that even when everything was checked, quality issues still surfaced. Members were confused, access broke down, financial stress increased, and trust eroded. And yet, when we looked back, all the boxes were marked complete. The work had been done, the process had been followed, and the checklist had been satisfied.

That was the moment I realized that **checking is necessary, but it is not sufficient**.

Healthcare quality professionals are often positioned as validators at the end of a process. We are brought in when decisions are already made, designs are largely finalized, and timelines are tight. Our role becomes one of confirmation rather than influence. We are asked to verify that things align with requirements, not to question whether those requirements truly protect people.

This positioning limits the impact of quality work, and it underestimates the responsibility we actually carry.

Over the years, I began to see quality not as a function, but as a form of guardianship. We are not just checking whether something is correct. We are guarding outcomes that people depend on, often without ever knowing our names. We are protecting access to care, financial safety, clarity, fairness, and trust. These are not abstract goals; they are lived experiences.

The difference between a checker and a guardian is not skill; it is mindset.

A checker asks, "Does this meet the requirement?"
A guardian asks, "What happens if this goes wrong?"
A checker looks for completion.
A guardian looks for consequences.

This shift does not happen automatically. It requires courage, curiosity, and a willingness to slow things down when the pressure is to move fast. It requires asking uncomfortable questions when confidence is high and time is short. And, it requires accepting that quality work will sometimes be invisible when done well—and highly visible when it is not.

One of the challenges quality professionals face is that success is often defined by absence. When nothing goes wrong, the work disappears into the background. When something does go wrong, quality is often asked why it wasn't prevented. This paradox can make the role feel thankless at times, but it also highlights how critical the role truly is.

I have seen quality professionals make the difference not by finding defects, but by asking the right questions early. Questions like: How will this feel to someone encountering it for the first time? What happens when timing doesn't align perfectly? Who is affected if this decision scales unexpectedly? What assumptions are we making about understanding, access, or resources?

These questions rarely show up on checklists, but they are often the ones that prevent harm.

"Quality is not about proving that something works.
It is about protecting people when it doesn't."

Becoming a guardian does not mean abandoning structure or discipline. It means expanding the purpose behind them. Requirements matter. Standards matter. Validation matters. But they are tools, not the destination. The destination is safe, fair, and understandable care.

The most effective quality professionals I have worked with understand this intuitively. They don't wait to be invited into conversations. They insert quality thinking where it matters most. They build relationships across teams. They translate technical decisions into human impact. And they advocate for people who are not in the room.

This role requires emotional intelligence as much as technical expertise. It requires the ability to navigate ambiguity, to communicate risk without alarm, and to balance progress with protection. It also requires humility, the recognition that no system is perfect and no design is final.

As healthcare continues to evolve, the need for quality guardians will only grow. Automation will accelerate decisions, complexity will increase, and pressure will intensify. In that environment, checkers will struggle to keep up. Guardians will shape the future.

As you reflect on your own role, consider where you currently operate. Are you primarily checking outputs, or are you guarding outcomes? Where could your questions prevent harm earlier? Where could your perspective add value before decisions harden?

This shift does not require a new title or authority. It begins with how you see your responsibility.

Because, when quality professionals embrace their role as guardians, healthcare becomes safer—not because systems are perfect, but because someone is watching over what truly matters.

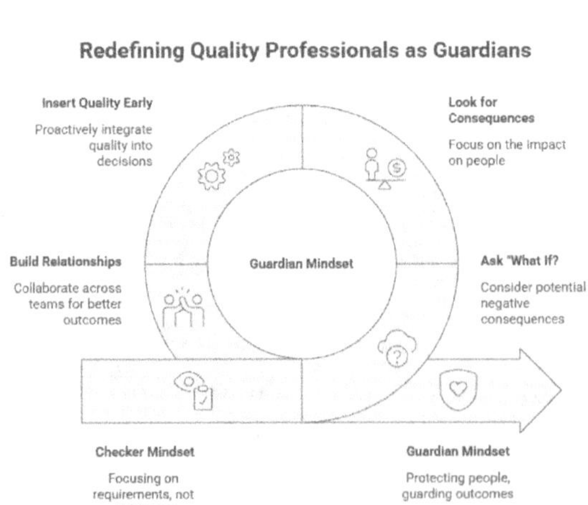
Redefining Quality Professionals as Guardians
Insert Quality Early
Proactively integrate quality into decisions
Look for Consequences
Focus on the impact on people
Build Relationships
Collaborate across teams for better outcomes
Guardian Mindset
Ask "What If?
Consider potential negative consequences
Checker Mindset
Focusing on requirements, not outcomes
Guardian Mindset
Protecting people, guarding outcomes

CHAPTER 15

Leading Quality: How Culture Shapes Outcomes Long Before Metrics Do

At some point in every healthcare quality journey, a realization settles in quietly: quality cannot be enforced into existence. It can be audited, measured, and reported, but it cannot be sustained unless the culture supports it. I have seen organizations with strong controls struggle because people felt unheard. I have seen others with fewer formal mechanisms succeed because quality was part of how decisions were made, not something applied afterward.

Leadership, in healthcare quality, is not about authority; it is about influence.

I used to believe that quality leadership meant having the right frameworks, escalation paths, and accountability structures. Those things matter, but they don't shape daily behavior nearly as much as how leaders respond to uncertainty, dissent, and mistakes. People watch closely what happens when someone raises a concern, challenges a decision, or admits a risk. Those moments teach more about quality than any policy ever will.

Culture is shaped in the space between intention and reaction. When leaders welcome questions, quality grows quietly. When leaders punish hesitation or rush for certainty, quality retreats. I have seen teams stop raising concerns not because risks disappeared, but because speaking up felt unsafe or futile. In those environments, issues don't vanish—they accumulate.

Quality culture is often misunderstood as compliance culture. In reality, the two can be at odds. Compliance focuses on adherence, quality focuses on understanding. A compliance-only culture asks, "Did we follow the rule?" A quality-driven culture asks, "Did we protect people?" The difference may seem subtle, but its impact is profound.

Research consistently shows that organizations with strong psychological safety report higher incident detection, faster learning cycles, and better long-term outcomes. That doesn't mean they make more mistakes—it means they see them sooner. In healthcare, early visibility is one of the strongest predictors of safety.

One of the most important lessons I have learned as a leader is that how we respond to bad news determines how much bad news we receive. When leaders react defensively or dismissively, people learn to filter what they share. When leaders respond with curiosity and accountability, people bring issues forward while they are still manageable.

"The culture of quality is revealed not when things go right, but when they don't."

Leading quality also requires consistency. Mixed signals are dangerous. When speed is rewarded publicly and caution is punished privately, quality becomes performative. Teams learn to say the right things while doing what they believe is actually expected. Over time, that disconnect erodes trust internally and externally.

Effective quality leaders align incentives with values. They recognize and reward thoughtful risk identification. They make space for reflection. They slow down when consequences matter. And they model the behavior they want others to adopt, not just in formal settings, but in everyday interactions.

Healthcare quality leadership is also deeply interdisciplinary. It requires collaboration across clinical, operational, technical, and administrative domains. Leaders who isolate quality within a single function limit its reach. Leaders who embed quality thinking across teams create resilience.

As healthcare becomes more complex and automated, the role of leadership becomes even more critical. Systems can process information, but they cannot set priorities or values. People do that. And people take cues from leadership, whether intentional or not.

I have learned that leading quality does not always mean being popular. It means being principled. It means asking hard questions when momentum is high. It means protecting long-term trust over short-term convenience.

And it means accepting that some of the most important quality work will never show up on a dashboard.

As you reflect on this chapter, consider how quality is modeled where you work. What behaviors are encouraged? Which ones are discouraged—explicitly or implicitly? How are concerns received? How are mistakes discussed?

Leadership is not limited to titles. Anyone who influences decisions, conversations, or norms is leading quality in some way.

The future of healthcare quality will not be determined by better tools alone. It will be determined by leaders, formal and informal, who choose to create environments where quality thinking can thrive.

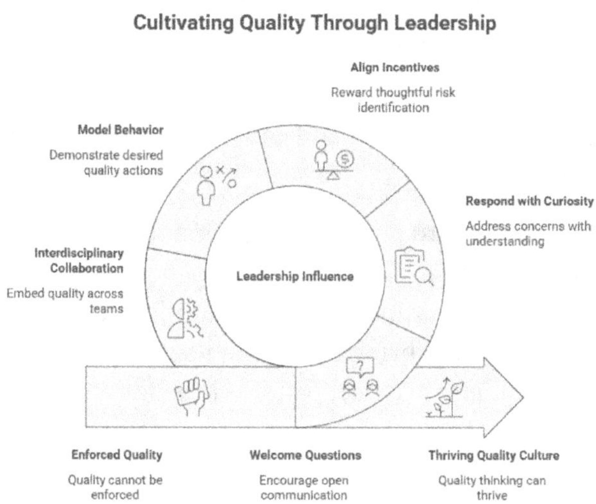
Cultivating Quality Through Leadership
Align Incentives
Reward thoughtful risk identification
Model Behavior
Demonstrate desired quality actions
Respond with Curiosity
Address concerns with understanding
Interdisciplinary Collaboration
Embed quality across teams
Leadership Influence
Enforced Quality
Quality cannot be enforced
Welcome Questions
Encourage open communication
Thriving Quality Culture
Quality thinking can thrive

CHAPTER 16

The Future of Healthcare Quality: Why Mindset Will Matter More Than Tools

Every era of healthcare believes it is on the edge of transformation. New technologies emerge, new models promise efficiency, and new metrics claim to measure what truly matters. And yet, across decades of change, one truth has remained consistent: systems evolve faster than our ability to understand their consequences fully.

As I look toward the future of healthcare quality, I am less concerned about whether we will have better tools and more concerned about whether we will use them wisely.

Healthcare is moving toward greater automation, more advanced analytics, and increasing reliance on artificial intelligence. Decisions that once required human review will increasingly be initiated, or even completed, by systems. This shift will bring real benefits: faster processing, greater consistency, and the ability to detect patterns humans might miss. But it will also amplify the consequences of poor assumptions and shallow thinking.

The future will not forgive quality failures simply because technology was involved.

One of the most important lessons I have learned is that complexity does not eliminate responsibility—it concentrates it. As systems become more powerful, the margin for error shrinks. A design flaw that once affected a handful of people may soon affect millions in a matter of hours. In that environment, quality professionals must think further ahead than ever before.

Research across healthcare and other high-reliability industries shows that technology-driven systems often outperform humans in stable, predictable environments, but struggle when context changes, data is incomplete, or values must be weighed. These are precisely the conditions that define healthcare. No algorithm can fully understand human fear, financial stress, or ethical nuance. Those remain human responsibilities.

This is where mindset becomes the defining factor.

Quality in the future will not be secured by adding more checkpoints or more controls. It will be secured by professionals who understand the system deeply, question assumptions continuously, and remain anchored in human impact. Tools can support that work, but they cannot replace it.

I believe the most successful healthcare quality professionals of the future will share a few defining traits. They will be systems thinkers who see beyond their immediate scope. They will be translators who can bridge technical, clinical, and human perspectives. They will be ethical stewards who recognize that speed, without care, creates risk. And they will be learners, constantly adapting as the system evolves.

"The future of quality will not be automated.
It will be guided."

Another important shift will be the growing expectation of transparency. People increasingly want to understand how decisions are made, not just what the outcome is. Trust will depend not only on correctness, but on explainability. Systems that cannot explain themselves clearly will struggle to maintain legitimacy, regardless of how accurate they are.

This places additional responsibility on quality professionals. We will be asked not only to validate outcomes, but to ensure that processes can be understood and defended in human terms. That is not a technical challenge; it is a communication and values challenge.

The future will also demand greater integration between quality, ethics and leadership. As decisions become faster and more complex, the ability to pause, reflect and ask, "Should we?" not just "Can we?" will distinguish safe systems from risky ones. That pause will rarely be built into technology. It must be built into culture.

As healthcare quality evolves, the temptation will be to chase the next innovation, the next framework, the next metric. Those things will continue to change. What must remain constant is the commitment to protect people, especially when systems are under pressure.

As I reflect on my own journey, what stands out is not the tools I have used or the processes I have mastered. It is the moments when someone asked a thoughtful question at the right time, the moments when quality slowed things down just enough to prevent harm, and the moments when mindset mattered more than momentum.

This book has argued one central idea from the beginning: quality is not a skillset. It is a mindset. Skills can be trained. Tools can be upgraded. Mindset determines how those skills and tools are used, especially when trade-offs are unavoidable.

As you reach the end of this book, I invite you to carry that mindset forward. Question assumptions, look beyond checklists, see the system, not just your part of it, and remember that behind every decision, every rule, and every process is a person depending on the system to behave responsibly.

The future of healthcare quality will be shaped not by technology alone, but by the people who choose to think deeply, act thoughtfully, and guard what truly matters.

That responsibility now belongs to you.

CHAPTER 17

Conclusion/Epilogue

Quality is the choice we make before anyone is watching.

As this book ends, I find myself returning to a simple truth that has followed me throughout my career in healthcare quality: the most important quality decisions are rarely the most visible ones. They are decisions made early, quietly, and often without recognition. They happen when no metric is flashing red, when no escalation has been raised, and when no one is yet feeling the impact.

Those decisions shape everything that follows.

Healthcare quality is often discussed as a function, a role, or a department. But in reality, it is a way of seeing. It is the ability to recognize how systems behave under pressure, how people navigate uncertainty, and how small assumptions can become large consequences. Quality is not something we add at the end of a process. It is something we carry with us into every decision we make.

Throughout this book, I have shared what I have seen, what I have learned, and what research continues to reinforce. I have seen systems that worked exactly as designed and still caused harm. I have seen people blamed for failures that were predictable outcomes of poor design. I have seen access delayed, trust eroded, and safety compromised—not because anyone intended it, but because quality thinking stopped too soon.

I have also seen the opposite. I have seen quality professionals slow things down just enough to ask better questions. I have seen leaders create space for uncertainty, instead of rushing for certainty. I have seen systems redesigned not for efficiency alone, but for clarity and fairness. And I have seen how those choices, often invisible, protected people in ways that never made headlines.

What connects all of these moments is mindset.

Skills matter. Tools matter. Frameworks matter. But mindset determines how those things are used when trade-offs are unavoidable. It determines whether speed overrides safety, whether compliance replaces understanding, and whether technology amplifies care or confusion. Mindset is what guides us when there is no clear answer, only responsibility.

"Quality is what remains when the checklist ends."

As healthcare continues to evolve, becoming faster, more automated and more complex, the need for a quality mindset will only grow. Technology will continue to change. Policies will shift. Metrics will evolve. But the human experience of healthcare will remain. People will still seek care during vulnerable moments. They will still depend on systems they do not fully understand. They will still feel the impact of decisions made far away from them.

Quality professionals stand at that intersection.

You may never meet the people you protect. You may never see the harm you prevent. And you may rarely receive credit for the outcomes you safeguard. But your influence is real. It lives in access that works, in clarity that reassures, in fairness that builds trust, and in systems that behave responsibly under pressure.

If there is one message I hope stays with you after reading this book, it is this: quality is not about perfection. It is about intention, awareness, and accountability. It is about choosing to see beyond your immediate task and recognizing the human consequences of your work. It is about guarding outcomes, not just validating processes.

Quality is not a skillset you master once.
It is a mindset you practice every day.

And, in healthcare, that mindset has the power to change lives—often without anyone ever knowing it was you.

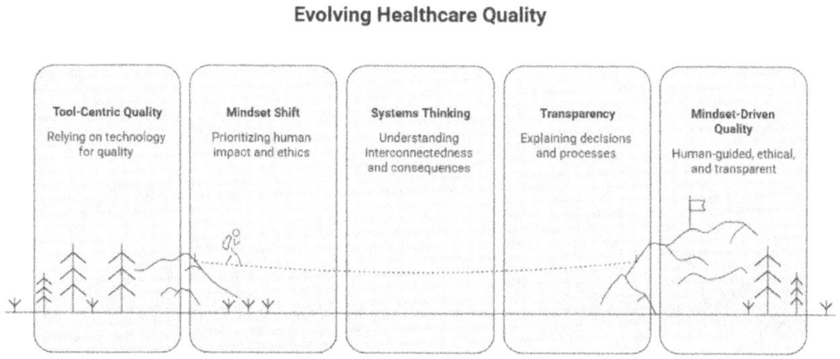
Evolving Healthcare Quality
Tool-Centric Quality
Relying on technology for quality
Mindset Shift
Prioritizing human impact and ethics
Systems Thinking
Understanding interconnectedness and consequences
Transparency
Explaining decisions and processes
Mindset-Driven Quality
Human-guided, ethical, and transparent

About the Author

Sravan Kumar Nidiganti has spent more than two decades working in environments where quality is not optional. His career began in highly regulated, safety-critical industries, where precision, validation, and disciplined execution were essential to protecting lives. Those formative experiences shaped his enduring belief that quality is not merely a task to complete, but a responsibility to advocate.

As he transitioned into healthcare and Pharmacy Benefit Management (PBM), that belief deepened. He witnessed firsthand how benefit accuracy, regulatory compliance, operational reliability, and data integrity directly influence patient access, affordability, and trust. To Sravan, healthcare quality is not abstract; it determines whether someone receives medication on time, understands their benefits, or can afford essential care.

Today, Sravan serves as a healthcare quality and operations leader, strengthening governance, implementing risk-based testing strategies, advancing automation, and integrating responsible AI across Medicare, Medicaid, EGWP, and Commercial populations. His work is centered on ensuring that healthcare systems operate accurately, ethically, and efficiently at scale.

As a Doctoral candidate in healthcare administration, Sravan embodies the scholar-practitioner model, bridging evidence-based quality frameworks with real-world operational execution. His research explores healthcare quality, patient safety, automation, and AI-enabled improvement—including robotic process automation in PBM quality assurance and the responsible application of AI in compliance-driven healthcare environments.

He is Six Sigma Green Belt certified, a Fellow of the American College of Health Data Management (ACHDM) and a Member of the American College of Healthcare Executives (ACHE). Sravan actively serves in leadership roles within the American Society for Quality (ASQ), contributes to professional forums, and speaks on healthcare quality, regulatory readiness, leadership, and emerging technologies. Beyond his professional commitments, he mentors students and healthcare professionals, encouraging them to lead with both empathy and accountability.

At the heart of his work lies a deep curiosity about access and affordability, how healthcare systems can reduce friction, improve clarity, and ensure that quality improvements translate into meaningful outcomes for patients and communities.

Through *Quality Is More a Mindset Than Skillset*, Sravan shares not only frameworks and strategies, but a philosophy: that true quality begins with values, is strengthened by discipline, and ultimately exists to serve people.

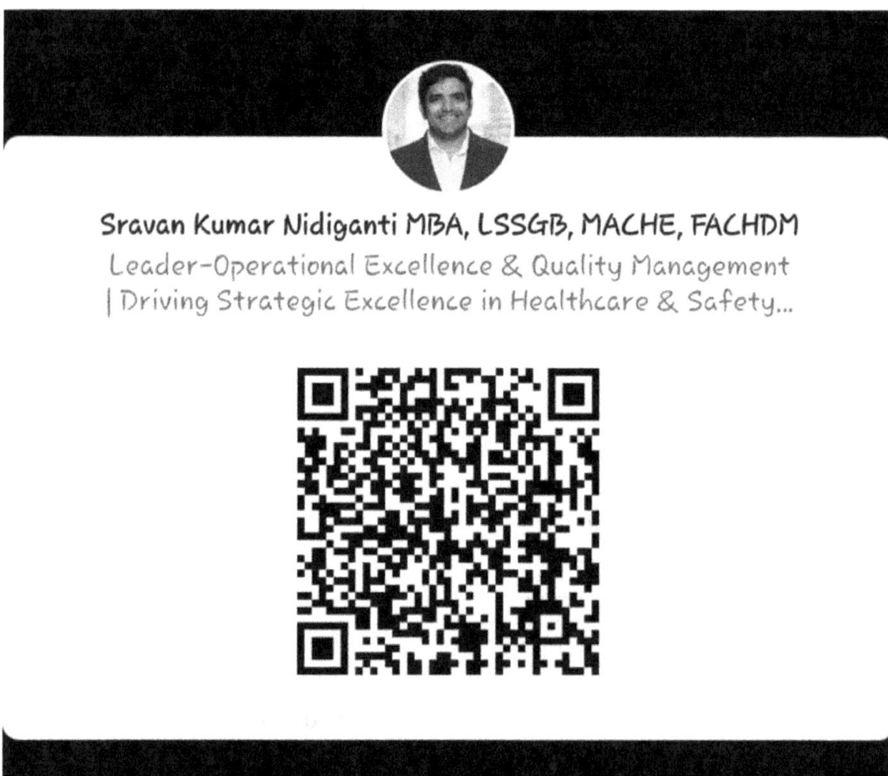
Sravan Kumar Nidiganti MBA, LSSGB, MACHE, FACHDM
Leader-Operational Excellence & Quality Management
| Driving Strategic Excellence in Healthcare & Safety...

www.ingramcontent.com/pod-product-compliance
Lightning Source LLC
LaVergne TN
LVHW022020200926
848481LV00007B/2463
9798903426812